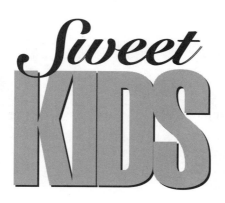

How to Balance Diabetes Control and Good Nutrition With Family Peace

BETTY PAGE BRACKENRIDGE, MS, RD, CDE

RICHARD R. RUBIN, PHD, CDE

PUBLISHER
Susan H. Lau

EDITORIAL DIRECTOR
Peter Banks

ACQUISITIONS EDITOR
Susan Reynolds

BOOK EDITOR
Karen Lombardi Ingle

DESKTOP PUBLISHER AND DESIGNER
Harlowe Typography, Inc.

ILLUSTRATOR
Timothy Cook

PRODUCTION DIRECTOR
Carolyn R. Segree

Library of Congress Cataloging-in-Publication Data

Brackenridge, Betty Page, 1943–
    Sweet kids : how to balance diabetes control and good nutrition
with family peace / Betty Page Brackenridge and Richard R. Rubin.
        p.   cm.
    ISBN 0-945448-67-8 (pbk.)
    1. Diabetes in children—Diet therapy.   2. Children—Nutrition.
I. Rubin, Richard R.   II. Title.
RJ420.B726   1996
    618.92'4620654—dc20   96-20277
                                                               CIP

American Diabetes Association, Inc.,
1660 Duke Street, Alexandria, VA 22314

Contents

CONTENTS

III Food, Diabetes, and Development

IV And Don't Forget to Take Care of You

Acknowledgments

• • • • • • • • • • • • • •

The following wonderful people—some health-care professionals and some parents of "sweet kids"—have reviewed our book. We thank them for their expertise and their time. Without them, we couldn't have produced the book you're holding.

JoAnn Ahern, RN, MSN, CS, CDE
New Haven, Connecticut

Jean Betschart, MN, RN, CDE
Pittsburgh, Pennsylvania

Keith Campbell, RPh, MBA, CDE
Pullman, Washington

Tess Curran
Phoenix, Arizona

Kim Heintzman, MS, RD, LD, CDE
Albuquerque, New Mexico

Ann Hussey
Wantagh, New York

Donna Jornsay, RN,CDE
Great Neck, New York

Gloria Loring
Los Angeles, California

Joyce Mosiman, RD, LD, CDE
Kansas City, Missouri

Joyce Green Pastors, RD, MS, CDE
Charlottesville, Virginia

Leslie Plotnick, MD
Baltimore, Maryland

Stephanie Schwartz, RN, MPH, CDE
Kansas City, Missouri

Susan Thom, RN, LD, CDE
Brecksville, Ohio

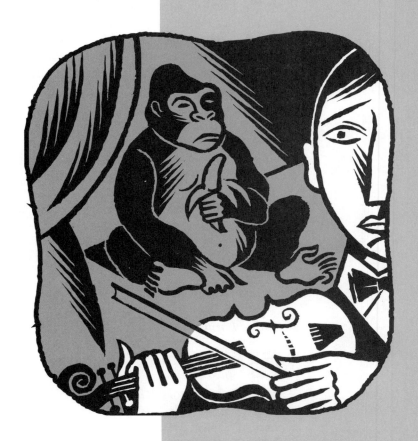

The gorilla at the symphony

BETTY PAGE BRACKENRIDGE

• • • • • • • • • • • • • •

What Diabetes Can Do to Families

Diabetes arrives on the scene like a gorilla at the symphony— impossible to ignore!

'd been in my first job as a dietitian only a few weeks when I got my first lesson in what diabetes can do to families. It came from Josh Taylor and his mother, Nancy. Josh was a handsome little 8-year-old with bright red hair and freckles. With his jeans, oversized striped T-shirt, and sneakers, he looked like the all-American boy. Mom, on the other hand, looked like a poster child for parental stress. She seemed worried and exhausted, with deep circles under her big blue eyes. Her mouth was a thin, tight line.

Josh's family had just enrolled in the health plan where I worked. Because Josh's growth had slowed down, the pediatrician sent him to see me so I could "adjust the calorie level" of his meal plan. The idea was to provide enough calories to get his growth back on track. But it soon became clear that the problem was much more complicated than an outgrown meal plan. In fact, Josh and his family were locked in mortal battle

1

over food up to six times a day. The struggles had been getting worse.

According to his mother, the amount of food on the meal plan was never quite right. Sometimes Josh wasn't very hungry. When that happened, Mom made him stay at the table until he cleaned his plate. She confessed that she hated to do it because it made him so unhappy, but she just couldn't think of any other way to get him to eat. Sometimes he would still be sitting at the dinner table when bedtime arrived.

She blushed and looked out my office window when she told me that she sometimes bribed Josh to finish a meal— offering extra allowance money, toys, and even movie tickets in exchange for a clean plate. She said this only happened when his blood sugar was really low before supper. She was just too frightened he'd have a severe low blood sugar reaction to not do something to get him to eat when he was already low.

Josh said he thought it was worse when he was still hungry after he finished eating. Sometimes he begged for more food, but his parents almost always refused. They believed they had to follow the meal plan to the letter for Josh's own good. They told him he could have "free" foods, like calorie-free gelatin or raw vegetables, if he was still hungry, since those wouldn't raise his blood sugar. But he usually refused and sulked until snack time.

They both agreed that the biggest battle of all happened when Mom found a stash of candy bars and snack cakes in an old shoe box in the back of Josh's closet. To hear them both talk about it, I'm sure the resulting blast must have been heard well above the Arizona state line, echoing through the red rock canyons of Utah and beyond.

I was dumbfounded by their troubles. My training hadn't prepared me to deal with what Josh and his family were going through. The family hadn't enjoyed a meal free of arguments and criticism in months. Josh bristled at every effort to control his food intake and was angry at his father and brother for eating the sweets he now was being denied.

These were nice, intelligent people doing their best to follow the doctor's orders. Mom and Dad felt they had to put the meal plan their previous doctor and dietitian had given them into action precisely as printed. Food choices, portions, and the timing of meals were all carefully laid out, but the struggle to follow the plan to the letter was taking a heavy toll on the family. And to make matters worse, all that effort and heartache didn't even keep Josh's blood sugar under control. He was having low blood sugars several times a week, his hemoglobin A_{1c} was 11.6%, and he had nearly stopped growing.

In the years since I first met Josh's family, I have learned a lot about the problems that can follow diabetes into the family circle. Shots may be frightening. Blood tests can be painful and expensive. Worries about complications are always somewhere in the background. But as hard as these things are, I believe food is often the most difficult thing for families to deal with. This is partly due to the fact that food can be an issue at almost any moment (not just two or three times a day, like shots and tests). Food has personal, cultural, and social meaning. That's why food issues can be highly emotional. As diabetes intrudes into this important area, arguments and decisions about food can affect every single day, confusing this developmentally critical area of family life.

After all, food is the very stuff of life. Receiving the right type and amount of food is essential to any young creature's growth from birth to maturity. The relationships and activities that surround eating give children their first lessons about life. In fact, food is such an important part of a child's experience, that pleasant or unpleasant eating and feeding can color his or her entire world. Food is intimately involved in physical, mental, and emotional development and, ultimately, in the child's successful growth into a separate and independent adult.

If a hungry infant is fed in a close and relaxed manner, she learns that the world is an okay place and that she can trust it. When feeding progresses normally, it helps the child learn to trust herself as well as the outside world. This happens as she begins to choose her own foods and to notice and respond to her body's signals of hunger and satisfaction. Decision-making, self-confidence, and positive self-image should all grow gradually at the family table.

These changes happen fairly smoothly when relaxed parents just do their job. Ideally, eating is handled in a matter-of-fact fashion. Mom and Dad put suitable foods on the table and model how people are expected to eat and behave themselves in their particular family. Each member eats according to his or her preferences and appetite in a friendly, low-key atmosphere. Foods are chosen not only for their nutritional properties, such as providing energy, vitamins, minerals, and protein, but also to add to the family's enjoyment and to express its preferences, culture, and environment. In addition, in a family that isn't obsessed with food, kids who aren't particularly hungry eat less than usual and then make up for it at the next meal. If they're terribly hungry, they eat more. No big deal.

But when diabetes arrives on the scene, like a gorilla at the symphony, it's impossible to ignore! Imagine what would happen if a great ape walked into a concert hall. As one musician and then another notices the gorilla, everything starts to fall apart. Music stands get knocked over. Nobody watches the conductor. The gorilla throws banana peels on the stage and grabs the wigs off the startled heads of well-dressed ladies. No more concert. Just a confused jumble of noise. People leave the concert hall with their minds in an uproar and the scent of bananas clinging to their clothes.

A silly picture, I agree. But it's also a pretty good image of what diabetes can do to the process of getting a family fed, nurtured, and civilized. Parents are driven to do difficult and sometimes painful things by their own worries and by health-care providers' expectations. They often try to control with a clock and a measuring cup what is meant to unfold naturally under the influence of each child's unique pattern of growth, development, and appetite. The normal progression of a child choosing his own food as he grows older may be drastically slowed or even stopped. Mom and Dad become the "food police." Power struggles follow. Families go to war over earth-shaking issues like how many vanilla wafers got eaten after school today. The effect on relationships, development, and stress levels can be overpowering.

But it is possible to regain sanity. Pleasant meals are not out of reach. Worries can be reduced. Sorry, they don't go away completely. A certain amount of worry just seems to go with the territory when you're a parent—diabetes or no diabetes.

Richard Rubin and I wrote this book to help families keep their sanity by handling food and diabetes with greater confidence and a measure of humor. We have done our best to make what we've written both practical and realistic. After all, you take care of a real family in the real world.

Throughout *Sweet Kids,* you'll find stories by and about families like yours. Some of them are funny. (It definitely helps to laugh.) Others are sad. (Sometimes crying can help, too.) But all are stories of the strength, creativity, wisdom, and love of families just like yours: families trying to live the best life possible while dealing with the realities of diabetes. Working with these families over the years has been both a privilege and the best schooling in the world. They've either taught us or driven us to learn literally everything you'll find in this book.

It's easy to gawk at the gorilla and forget the symphony. It's also easy to become so focused on diabetes that your child's personal needs, as well as your own, never get proper attention. If the joy of eating and preparing food has disappeared, if spontaneity seems to be lost forever, or if you're just looking for some new ideas on how to cope with food and diabetes, please read on.

RICHARD R. RUBIN

When It's Your Child With Diabetes

I felt overwhelmed, and I desperately wanted not to feel that way.

April 2, 1979. I sat with my 7-year-old son Stefan as his pediatrician confirmed what I had suspected for the past few weeks: Stefan had diabetes. The signs had been there. The nearly nonstop drinking, the equally constant urination, the tremendous hunger, and the home urine glucose test that read 4+. Back then, 17 years ago, the only way we could test for sugar at home was by testing urine. Blood sugar testing didn't arrive until a couple of years later.

As we sat there listening to Doctor Bill tell us all the ways in which our lives were about to change, I felt nervous, even downright scared. My thoughts returned to a day almost exactly 20 years earlier when my sister Mary Sue, then 9 years old, was diagnosed with diabetes. Her diabetes had been hard for my family. We didn't talk about it much. But, in a way, that only made it seem worse. I could see her stress as she tested, gave herself shots with those old glass syringes that had to be boiled before each use, sharpened the needles so her shots wouldn't hurt so much,

6

and make all the myriad daily adjustments that were now a part of her life.

I could also see the pressure diabetes placed on my parents. They worked hard to make sure that, among other things, she ate *exactly* the right amount of *exactly* the right foods at *exactly* the right time. They did a good job, but making that happen meant that life was very tightly structured at our house, once diabetes had arrived.

Those memories and much more darted through my mind on that early April morning. I felt overwhelmed, and I desperately wanted not to feel that way. I wanted to feel strong. I wanted to feel confident that Stefan and I and the whole family could take diabetes in stride, that we could cope, that our lives could remain wonderful. But I had my doubts. I needed to see a ray of light, and I found one right at hand. Doctor Bill, having finished his description of Stefan's diabetes care regimen, turned to me and said, "Okay, Dick, now you pull down your pants. I want you to stick yourself with this syringe to show Stefan that it doesn't hurt too much." Down as I had been feeling, this crazy thought went through my mind: "At least I'm wearing clean underwear."

Then I laughed for the first time in what must have been weeks. I told Bill and Stefan what I'd been thinking, and they laughed, too. The tension eased for all of us, and my confidence that we could cope was restored. Naturally, this was only the first step on the very long and never-ending road that all families living with diabetes must travel. But it was a crucial step, nonetheless. I believed we could manage, even before I knew exactly what we would have to do or how we would do it.

From the moment Stefan's diabetes was diagnosed, I tried to learn as much as I could about his disease and its management. I talked to Stefan's team and lots of other diabetes health-care providers. I read lots of books. We received instruction and attended classes. They all kept coming back to the same point: "If your child eats right, exercises, and takes his insulin, he (and you) can lead a perfectly normal life." Much as I wanted to believe these encouraging words, experience quickly taught me they simply weren't true. That's not to say our life was bleak, because it wasn't. It was still wonderful, full, and exciting. In many ways, it was even more exciting than it had been before diabetes. But normal it wasn't and still isn't.

How can life be normal with all the planning and adjusting, worrying and readjusting that are a continuing fact of life with diabetes? The planning, worrying, and adjustments are facts of life for both managing the diabetes regimen and fitting that regimen into the rest of your family's life—or what's left of that life after diabetes becomes a daily reality. Many parents say that the early stages of life with diabetes remind them of what it was like to have a new baby. Among other things, you've always got to carry stuff with you to deal with potential emergencies. Only now, instead of toting bottles and diapers and baby wipes, it's snacks and syringes, insulin and blood glucose meters.

Many of the adjustments you make when your child gets diabetes are food-related. That's not surprising, since food and eating touch every waking moment. Food is different from other aspects of diabetes care. Once your child has taken his shot or tested his blood glucose, no one needs to worry about those things until the next time. The same is true of exercise. But at any moment of the day, your child can eat too much or too little, or eat the wrong things. Moreover, eating is something everyone does, so his eating has to somehow fit with what the rest of your family is doing.

In the first months after Stefan's diabetes was diagnosed, we worked hard to get his eating just right. We weighed and measured and struggled to memorize the American Dietetic Association and American Diabetes Association's *Exchange Lists*. Looking back, I see that all of this was helpful. It gave us a solid foundation on which to build our own unique structure for life with diabetes—a structure that suited our lifestyle and our son's need to grow up as healthy and normal as possible.

Since 1979, I've worked with many families who are living with diabetes, and I've learned from every one of them. The families have taught me how powerfully having a child with diabetes can affect family life. My work has also taught me how creatively and beautifully some families manage that challenge. And, perhaps most important of all, I've learned how some of these families who do so well manage to do it. The guidelines and suggestions offered in this book are drawn from that experience. In *Sweet Kids*, Betty Brackenridge and I share with you all the practical lessons we have learned over the years.

My greatest teacher is still my son Stefan. He is living proof that it is possible to grow up healthy and strong with diabetes. May your child flourish as wonderfully as he has.

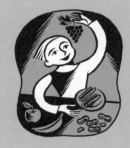

The first section
of the book
summarizes what
experts know about
feeding kids right.
Not just children
with diabetes. All
kids.

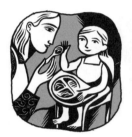

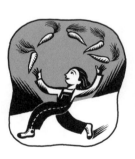

Healthy Eating and Feeding for All Families

The first section of the book summarizes what experts know about feeding kids right. Not just children with diabetes. All kids. The fact that your child has diabetes does not change his or her basic needs—either nutritionally or emotionally.

Helping your child internalize control over food choices and amounts is an important key to lifelong health and better diabetes control. In Chapter 1, we describe the best approach we know of to help your child develop that internal control.

Chapter 2 covers the body's natural system for appetite regulation in detail and describes how to make sure your child is eating the right amount of food. In Chapter 3, we talk about the kinds of foods that you and your child with diabetes need to stay healthy. We review why eating well has become something of a struggle for most people and exactly what's involved in making good food choices.

Throughout the book we'll be describing ways to fine-tune food, insulin, and exercise to promote more stable and desirable blood sugar control. But those tricks won't work very well until the basics are right—the right amount of food for the child's needs and the right amount of insulin to allow the body to use that amount of food.

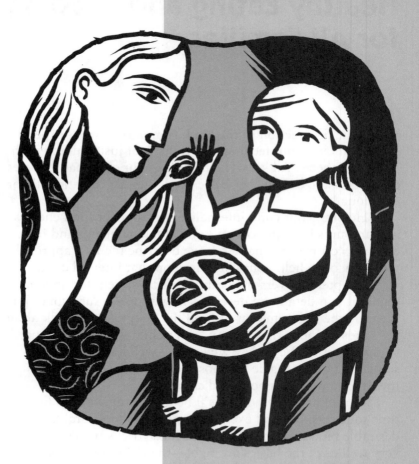

• • • • • • •

"It seemed that the more I forced, the less she ate..."

What Parents Can Do to Promote Healthy Eating

The older the baby got, the more creative she became at avoiding unwanted food.

Picture 15-month-old Lucy and her mother in their cheerful yellow kitchen. Ginger, the baby's mother, has spread a big blue shower curtain under the highchair and covered the stove top and canister set with plaid dish towels. She's wearing her husband's barbecue apron over her clothes. Lucy is stripped down to the bare essentials: diaper and bib. It's time for lunch, and it isn't going to be pretty.

When Lucy developed diabetes at 8 months of age, she was eating rice cereal and milled carrots eagerly and still being breast-fed. As Lucy's mother described those past mealtimes, her face lit up with a big grin. Nursing had created islands of calm in their busy days. She and Lucy cheerfully snuggled through most feedings, unaware of their surroundings. As for solid foods, Ginger said, "Sometimes Lucy didn't eat a whole lot, but she always smiled and chattered at me. I could tell when she'd had enough because she'd clamp the spoon

13

between her gums and give me a wicked little smile." That was before diabetes.

The first big change had been to do away with breast-feeding. The dietitian said there was no way to tell if Lucy was taking in enough when she breast-fed. Formula out of a bottle would be "much easier to keep track of." Reluctantly, Lucy's mom agreed, but the transition hadn't been easy. It was one more change to deal with at an already difficult time. Insulin shots, blood glucose testing, worry, grief. It had all been so hard. "Someday I'll write a book," she told me.

Each feeding consisted of a certain number of ounces of formula and one or two servings of cereal, fruit, vegetables, or meat. Ginger dutifully began trying to make Lucy eat it all. But the more she forced, the less Lucy ate. Their struggle escalated as Mom got more and more desperate. The baby responded by going on the offensive. The fur (and food) began to fly. Until Ginger thought of using that shower curtain to catch the overflow, she had been washing the floor, walls, and counters after every meal.

Lucy still clamped her jaw down when she'd had enough. But now, instead of letting it slide, her mother would try various tricks to get those last few bites down the reluctant baby's throat. She'd begin with the make-believe choo-choo train or airplane deliveries of baby food. Eventually, she'd sink to prying the child's mouth open and shoveling the food in while Lucy struggled. The older the baby got, the more creative and experienced she became at avoiding unwanted food. Spitting, spilling, throwing, smearing: she became a true artist at keeping the offending items from reaching her stomach. Ginger swore that Lucy stayed cheerful about the whole situation. But Mom wasn't in the same frame of mind.

"I'm not sure that it's worth the struggle," she said. "Her blood sugars are a mess anyway. I'm tempted to just forget the whole thing: to let Lucy eat what she wants and then try to keep up with it as best I can."

Ginger was frustrated and exhausted. Even so, she and Lucy were doing much better than a lot of families. What made the difference was the fact that Lucy was keeping her cool. That's not usually the case in situations like this.

The more common result when children are forced to eat is that they become angry and combative. Their anger—perhaps acted out complete with crying, screaming, squirming, and other thoroughly unattractive behaviors—often makes parents force even harder, and the war escalates. "Eat it or else!" "You can't leave the table till all those noodles are gone!" It's no fun. And a no-win game for all concerned. These battles seldom produce the desired effect. When the smoke clears, not only is the food not eaten, but everybody is irritated as well.

DO YOU KNOW YOUR JOB DESCRIPTION?

Like the food battles just described, Lucy's balky response to her mom's strong-arm tactics was predictable. It happened because Mom overstepped the bounds of her job description. You may not believe that there are clearly defined food-related job descriptions for parents and kids, but there are. And while you usually don't see them written down anywhere, they are still very real. Trouble almost always results when those roles aren't played out as they should be.

What those roles involve in the area of food and feeding is nicely summarized in an old cliché: "You can lead a horse to water, but you can't make him drink." Simply put, parents are supposed to provide the food. Kids then decide whether or not to eat it. We know this may sound unreasonable, and even unsafe, at first, especially in light of advice you may have gotten from other health-care providers. Letting children follow their appetites may sound suspect because of your own childhood experiences, or because of your concerns about high and low blood sugars. But helping your child internalize control over food choices and amounts is an important key to lifelong health and better diabetes control.

Hunger and thirst are internal: internal to horses at watering troughs and internal to children at the dinner table—in fact, internal to us all. No one can tell from the outside whether a child is hungry or thirsty on the inside—not a well-meaning parent and certainly not a doctor or dietitian sitting in an examination room miles from home. It's true that kids eventually get old enough to tell us these things. But unfortunately, even when they do tell us, we sometimes ignore them.

"I'm full, Mom," declares your pride and joy. "Aw, c'mon, Jeffrey. Clean up your plate. I fixed it just for you!" Our intentions are good. We want our children to eat enough, to eat the right things, and—maybe just once in a while—to get really full so they don't bug us for a snack during the Saturday afternoon movie.

At one time or another, nearly all parents (with or without the unique pressures of diabetes) attempt to control how much their children eat by either forcing or withholding food. Their parents did it to them. And they're passing on the favor to the next generation. What can it hurt to encourage, pressure, or even browbeat the kids to eat? It sounds simple and logical. They need food. We make sure they eat it. And we're bigger than they are. It shouldn't be so tough.

FORCING CHILDREN TO EAT DOESN'T WORK

Forcing children to eat is tough because it violates a perfectly good internal system of control that we are all programmed to develop. Trying to force a child who isn't hungry to eat is very much like trying to force a lively child to go to sleep. It almost never works. If you're lucky, the little jumping bean eventually falls asleep because she's exhausted from bouncing in and out of bed, sneaking down the hall, and so on. And your reluctant eater will eat sooner or later, mostly because you've been fighting for so long that she finally becomes hungry. But forcing the issue usually produces an angry or beaten child who actually ends up eating *less* than she would have if left alone. And it wears out the parents.

Cleaning up your plate has been a big issue between parents and children for a very long time. Even though we are approaching the end of the century, many parents and grandparents are still affected by memories of the Great

Depression of the 1930s. They either lived through it themselves or were raised by people who remember those hard years when food was scarce and precious. It was important to eat everything you could when food was available. The truth was that it might not be around if you waited until later to eat. And so, at least since the Depression ended, American children have been urged repeatedly and forcefully to "clean up that plate" when a few peas or half of a lamb chop were still hanging around at the end of the meal.

Many methods have been used to enforce the clean plate policy. Some of us were told how much the food had cost our hard-working parents. Others got the philosophical party line, "Waste not, want not." Countless kids heard about the plight of the poor starving children in (depending on generation) Poland, China, Bangladesh, Ethiopia, and now, perhaps, Rwanda. And a myriad of moppets were simply left to stew in their juices at the kitchen table until late into the night— "You're not leaving this table until you eat that perfectly good liver and Brussels sprouts!"

One unintended but very real effect of that kind of pressure is to teach kids to ignore or doubt what their own bodies are telling them. A child may say to himself, "Gee, I feel full, but Mom says I should eat more. Maybe I should ignore what I feel. After all, she's Mom, and I'm just a kid. She probably knows best." This is one reason why some adults have trouble controlling their food intake. They never learned to eat when they're hungry and then stop when they're full. Instead, they tend to eat because of things outside themselves—the time of day, the presence of food, social pressure, the desire to please others, and so on.

WITHHOLDING FOOD FROM HUNGRY KIDS DOESN'T WORK EITHER

Today, parental pressure about food often takes the opposite form: withholding food when kids are still hungry. The main reason for this seems to be the immense value that our culture places on being thin. As a result, parents can be tempted or even encouraged by physicians (we're sorry to say) to place children on diets. This is a more risky and complicated issue than it seems to be at first glance. If you are concerned about weight, weight loss, or body type in your children, we urge you to read *How To Get Your Kids To Eat...But Not Too Much* by Ellyn Satter (Bull Publishing, Palo Alto, CA, 1987) for some excellent practical advice.

Diabetes seems to encourage both types of controlling behavior. Parents sometimes feel compelled to make their children eat more in order to cover their insulin. At other times, they worry that children are eating too much, which might raise blood sugar, and so they try to stop the kids from eating all they want. Trying to manage food in these ways seems logical, but it doesn't work in the long run.

FOLLOW THE JOB DESCRIPTION TO REACH LONG-TERM GOALS

If parents persist too long in controlling food choices and amounts eaten, children have a hard time learning to internalize control over their food intake. This goal is important for both the child and the parent. After all, if your child doesn't learn to manage her own food intake, one day you may have to get day passes from the old folks' home to make sure that your elderly "baby" is cleaning up her plate!

All joking aside, if there's one thing that's vital to the child with diabetes, it's learning to manage food successfully. She'll need that skill all her life to feel well and stay healthy. She won't get to that point if you control choices and portions until she's 18 and then say, "Now it's your job, dear." The process starts in infancy (remember Lucy) and proceeds through predictable stages until—voilà—she stands before you one day able to manage her own nutrition. Babies, toddlers, and preschool-age children begin to learn food patterns and preferences as they pick and eat their fill from the good foods their parents provide. School-age children choose, sometimes wisely, sometimes not, from the wider variety of foods available outside the family home. And finally, teenagers become able to plan meals for themselves and others, hopefully without dooming anyone to scurvy or a heart attack. Not that they'll do these things perfectly at any stage. But they will be capable of making their own choices and, eventually, of doing at least as good a job as the rest of us.

IGNORING JOB DESCRIPTIONS CAN HARM FAMILY RELATIONSHIPS

Trying to control your child's food intake too closely puts you and your child on opposite sides in a negative and painful battle. You become the "food police." And like the wonderful little rebels that they are, kids rise to the challenge. Arguments over food strain your relationship just when you most need to stand united in dealing with diabetes. There is a better way. And that is for everyone involved to know and follow their job description.

THE PARENTS' JOB DESCRIPTION

In feeding their children, parents are responsible for only four things:

1. Get the right foods on the table. The right foods are the kinds you want the kids to eat. Choose a variety of healthful foods (see Chapter 3 for details on choosing the right foods for the whole family's health). Prepare foods or buy them prepared. Get the kids to help with preparation according to their age and ability. Remember, if they cut the carrots, they'll be more interested in eating them! Get those good foods onto the table or lunch counter or into the lunch box. No fuss. No PR job ("Oh, yum, Brussels sprouts!"). Just get them out there. Too much hype over the more healthful choices you want to encourage will just make kids suspicious. After all, no one gives them a sell job for things like french fries and brownies. You can't fight the logic, "If those Brussels sprouts were so great, would she really need to sell them so hard?" Away from home, children will be exposed to lots of less healthy choices, especially as they get older. But being offered mostly healthy foods at home from a young age helps your child develop preferences for those better choices. He still won't always make great choices when he's away from your watchful eye. But he'll make *more* good choices than he would if you hadn't exposed him to the right stuff to begin with.

2. Make family meals regular, peaceful, and important. Have regular meals at which family members are expected to show up, eat as much as they want of what's offered, and allow everyone else to do the same. Regular meals are needed, because kids need frequent feeding. Of course, this becomes even more important when diabetes enters the picture.

Today, more and more families are eating separately on the fly instead of sitting down to meals together. Try to fight the trend. We know that eating every meal together is an unrealistic goal for most families. Individual schedules and responsibilities may make it difficult. But do the best you can, because it's really important.

Family meals are where children learn not only *what* to eat but also *how* to eat it. Manners, managing knife and fork, how to act when faced with a new or disliked food; these are important social skills. Eating alone in front of the TV or out of a box does not produce a socially competent person. We're assuming you want your children to learn their table manners and food preferences from you—not from the other second graders in the cafeteria or from the food ads on TV.

The only way we know to shape children's food preferences and manners in the direction parents prefer is to eat together regularly. Another problem that can play havoc with family meals occurs when mealtimes are used to argue, criticize, or hash out major conflicts. Again, don't do it. The result will be indigestion and a lot of negative associations around food and eating. Catch up on everybody's news. Hand out praise. Plan for the weekend. But keep mealtimes pleasant, so everyone can eat in peace.

3. Eat what you want your children to eat. Eating what you want your children to eat is a challenge for many parents, but it eliminates a great deal of hassle. Children learn their nutritional habits the way they learn language, values, and much more: by observation. "Do as I say, not as I do," isn't nearly as effective as, "This is the way we do it in our family."

Healthy eating for your child with diabetes is the same as it is for all members of the family. And new knowledge about sweets and diabetes makes it easier than you think for everyone in the family to be on the same nutritional wavelength.

Try not to single out your child with diabetes for what will surely be seen as the "punishment" of eating a variety of healthful foods while parents, brothers, or sisters eat differently. Forcing the child with diabetes to eat quite differently from other family members is also bound to create problems and resentments.

Instead, use diabetes as an opportunity to improve everyone's health. Good nutrition is the cornerstone of good health. The right foods fuel an active life and keep illness to a minimum. These are not benefits that should be reserved only for the family member with diabetes. Everyone in the family will benefit from a sensible approach to fat in the diet, and no one ought to be gorging on sweets.

It's possible to find a healthful, rational, and *enjoyable* approach to nutrition that fits the whole family's needs.

4. Stay in charge, even if the fur starts to fly! You choose and prepare the food, and you set the mealtime rules. Sometimes, children will question those choices and challenge the rules. That's to be expected. When it happens, stick by your guns with as much calm as you can muster. Children need to know what to expect. Be firm and consistent. It's not helpful to the family, to the child, or even to ongoing diabetes control to let short-term concerns about blood sugar disrupt the reassuring and predictable flow of family love or discipline.

THE CHILD'S JOB DESCRIPTION

Children are responsible for two things:

1. Decide how much to eat of the available foods. Have faith. Children don't voluntarily starve themselves. When they're hungry, they eat. And what's more, if left to their own devices, the vast majority of children even eat the right amount for their needs.

2. Follow family rules for mealtime behavior. Part of your job as a parent is making sure that mealtimes are pleasant for everyone—you included. This means that you will have expectations or rules for acceptable mealtime behavior. These rules will include things like sitting in your chair while you're eating, not throwing food, not yelling. The particulars depend, to a great extent, on your own style and on your children's ages. Are your family meals casual or do mater and pater "dress" for dinner? Are fingers acceptable utensils or is everyone over the age of 2 expected to use knife and fork? Whatever your rules are, the children need to observe them. When they don't do so after a couple of reminders, it's okay to ask them, firmly and calmly, to leave the table so everyone else can eat in peace. Not setting and enforcing rules may make it easier for children to use their diabetes to manipulate you and the rest of the family.

We know that this system can sound frightening to the parents of a child with diabetes, but it's the best approach we know. And it does work. It is possible to keep your child with diabetes safe and shape his or her good lifetime eating habits without creating major power struggles over food. You may win a battle or two when you try to micromanage your child's food intake. But don't let those occasional triumphs fool you. You are in a war that cannot be won. If you're interested in avoiding food fights and in helping your children learn to choose foods wisely and control their own intake, follow the parent and child job descriptions.

THE BOTTOM LINE

- Forcing children to eat doesn't work.
- Withholding food from hungry kids doesn't work, either.
- To avoid fights and help children develop internal control over food intake, follow the job descriptions:

The Parents' Job Description

1. Get the right foods on the table.
2. Make family meals regular, peaceful, and important.
3. Eat what you want your children to eat.
4. Stay in charge, even if the fur starts to fly!

The Child's Job Description

1. Decide how much to eat of the available foods.
2. Follow family rules for mealtime behavior.

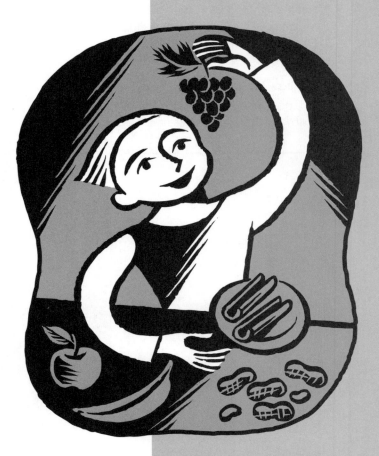

"He's got such a huge appetite, I'm afraid he'll get fat..."

How to Tell if He's Eating the Right Amount

Brandon was about average height for a 3-year-old and as solid as a brick wall. He was the most active little guy you can imagine: a living study in perpetual motion. He didn't just walk, he trotted or ran everywhere. He didn't just hug you when he burst through the office door, he launched himself straight into your arms. His dad pronounced him to be "All boy and a yard wide," which seemed an understatement to us all.

He was obviously thriving, but his eating was worrying his mother nearly to death. "How can he eat so much?" she asked. "The dietitian gave us a 1,200-calorie meal plan, but he's never satisfied with that. He gets angry when I won't let him have another piece of bread or more cereal. When I tell him he has to wait until snack time, he throws a fit. I try to fill him up with carrot and celery sticks, but he's back demanding more in no time. Tell me what I can do about his appetite. He can't go on eating twice as much as the other 3-year-olds and not turn into a butterball!"

It looked to us like Brandon probably needed exactly what his body was telling him to eat. We suggested a trial of putting the food on the table and letting Brandon eat as much as he liked, while keeping track of it all. We would help with insulin adjustments over the phone, if necessary. But we wanted to see exactly what Brandon's appetite urged him to eat. We were pretty sure that his weight wouldn't be a problem and that his diabetes control could be worked around his very healthy appetite. We also suspected that if Mom stopped trying to restrict his intake, he wouldn't be quite so desperate about it. All of that proved to be the case.

Over the years, we have suggested to many parents that they stop trying to control how much their children eat. It's seldom been a popular suggestion. Some of these folks have been pressuring their children to eat almost since they first coaxed a nipple into the baby's mouth. Others have been withholding food. Like Brandon's mom, they are confident that they know, better than the child, how much he should eat. The prospect of sitting back and letting Nature take its course usually makes them very nervous. Those in the first group worry that if they stop urging their children to eat, the kids will stop eating altogether. The others are sure that their kids, if left on their own, will never stop eating.

But those things almost never happen. There are exceptions, of course (see Chapter 9). Just how is the appetite regulating system supposed to work? Under natural conditions, people eat when they're hungry and stop when they're full. The amount of food that their own body tells them to eat is the right amount to maintain their natural body type: whether it is average or heavy, muscular or slim. This system can be sidetracked by certain conditions. But when everything's operating as it should, appetite is extremely well-tuned to calorie needs.

We know it's hard to believe, especially in our calorie-conscious society, but it's true. You can look to Nature to build a little confidence in this system before you try it. To begin with, we know that obesity almost never exists in animals living a natural existence. Even when the African veldt is absolutely lousy with antelope, lions maintain a normal lion weight. They eat to satisfy their hunger. When they're not hungry, they lie around in the shade, explore the territory, teach the kids how to stalk, and generally live the lion good life.

Of course, there are important differences between the lions' situation and our own. For one thing, there are no couch-potato lions. Lions have to run around—a lot—to get lunch. Also, TV remote controls are unknown on the veldt, no one has begun to market deep-fried antelope with sour cream dipping sauce to the lions, and the king of beasts does not eat chocolate when he's under stress. Unfortunately, these conditions are known to us (and to our children), and they can get in the way of normal appetite and weight regulation. But in most cases, people who are active, who eat a variety of healthful foods, and who follow the dictates of their own appetite regulate naturally to their own appropriate weight without counting a single calorie.

This system breaks down when people are very inactive, which is undoubtedly a major factor in the increase in obesity that we have seen in recent years. Our bodies weren't designed to be plopped down for hours every day in front of a TV or computer screen. Our ancestors had to be physically active to survive, so our bodies are suited to an active lifestyle. When we're not active, things get out of balance. We gain weight, and our appetite gets out of sync with our energy needs. We have to try to control from the outside (with willpower and brainpower) what was meant to be naturally regulated from the inside. It doesn't work very well, as evidenced by our huge and ineffective weight-loss industry. If you can get your kids up off the couch and onto their bikes or the playground, you greatly increase the chances that their appetite will match what they really need. That will make sticking to a well-designed meal plan or pattern much easier.

Add to the fact that overeating is very uncommon in nature the fact that starvation is never self-imposed. In the animal kingdom, starvation is only seen when there isn't enough food available. Deer starve in a drought year because their food supply disappears, not because the mother deer neglected to urge Bambi to crop off all the leaves in the clearing. Human beings can and do operate by this same system. For most of us, then, hunger is the best guide to how much food to eat. Satisfaction tells us when we've had enough.

Maybe you're thinking that this is all very well and good for other kids, but that diabetes changes the rules. While it's true that there are many things that diabetes changes, energy needs is not one of them. *Diabetes doesn't affect how much food your child needs.* Energy (calorie) needs depend on body size, growth rate, metabolic rate, how much exercise (play) the child gets (a big factor in Brandon's case), and other factors. Energy requirements vary a lot from child to child and even from day to day in the same child. The trick is to make sure that the child with diabetes eats the right amount, and then provide the right amount of insulin to allow his body to use that food for growth and energy needs.

The reliability of the internal system for regulating food intake is now well-recognized by scientists, even for children with diabetes. That recognition has only come about fairly recently, and so not all health-care providers are aware of it yet. For a long time, most diabetes meal plans were developed by calculating a calorie level based on weight. The dietitian or doctor consulted a chart or punched a few numbers into a calculator and said, "1,500 calories," or some other nice, round, specific number. The child with diabetes was then expected to eat just that much every day: no more, no less.

Those calculated calorie levels were almost never exactly right, and often they were actually way off base. It's not easy to accurately predict a given person's calorie needs. Body size is only one factor. Activity level and metabolic rate are also extremely important. For example, researchers have shown that big, heavy babies actually eat less (on average) than small, wiry infants who tend to be more active. Are heavy babies less active because they're heavy, or are they heavy because they're inactive? Maybe they're heavy and inactive because it's their nature. No one knows for sure. But we do know that there's no way to precisely predict a given person's energy (calorie) needs. However, when the internal appetite regulation system operates naturally, it is extremely precise and it adjusts automatically for growth and activity. The body can be more exact than any dietitian with a calculator.

And being exact is very important. Every extra calorie will be stored as body fat. (For example, just one extra Starch serving per day over actual calorie needs will add about 8 pounds in a year.) And every calorie that's missing is withheld from some needed body process.

BASE MEAL PLANS ON USUAL EATING HABITS

Calculating a prescribed calorie level is no longer considered the best way to design a meal plan in type I diabetes. Rather, the latest nutrition recommendations of the American Diabetes Association direct health-care providers to base the meal plan on an assessment of each person's "usual eating habits," and then match the insulin to that pattern. This new guideline expresses confidence in each person's internal system for regulating appetite and weight. If your child's weight is already in a desirable range, then the amount he's been eating is right for him. It makes much more sense to find out what that amount is and then base his diabetes meal plan on that rather than starting from scratch with a calculated plan that may or may not be right. If your child's weight is above or below a desirable range, his food intake, activity, and eating behavior all need to be closely reviewed to see if there is a problem and to determine how to best deal with it.

Basing the diabetes meal plan on a child's existing eating pattern also acknowledges the fact that diabetes management, in order to be successful, must be tailored as much as possible to the real circumstances of the person's life. Building the meal plan around the family's actual schedule, lifestyle, and food preferences makes it more likely that the family and the child will be able to follow it.

To make this approach work, expect the dietitian to ask you to keep good records of what your child eats and drinks for a period of from 3 days up to a week. The dietitian will then

TABLE 2.1 Carbohydrate Counting Meal Plan Based on Usual Intake

	Lucy's Food Record	Carbohydrate Count Meal Plan	
Meal or Snack	Food Eaten and Amount	Carbohydrate/ Item g	Total Carbohydrate g
Breakfast	1/2 cup milk	6	
	1/4 cup rice baby cereal	10	
	1/3 cup orange juice	10	
	1 scrambled egg	0	~25
Morning Snack	1/3 cup milk	4	
	1 zweiback	5	~10
Lunch	1/2 cup milk	6	
	1/3 slice wheat toast with	5	
	2 tsp. peanut butter	0	
	1/4 ripe banana	8	~20
Afternoon Snack	1/2 cup milk	6	
	2 arrowroot cookies	9	~15
Dinner	1/2 cup milk	6	
	1/4 cup oat baby cereal	10	
	1 soda cracker	3	
	2 tbs. cooked carrots	2	
	2 tbs. applesauce	4	~25
Bedtime Snack	1/3 cup milk	4	
	1 zweiback	5	
	2 baby sausages	0	~10

analyze those records to determine the number of calories and amount of carbohydrate eaten and the usual pattern of meals and snacks throughout the day. A basic meal plan will be drawn up that expresses your child's usual eating pattern in terms of a specific meal planning system, such as exchanges or carbohydrate counting (more on this in Chapter 5). The things that make up your child's insulin regimen—types of insulin, number of injections, dose amounts, and timing—can be chosen to get the best possible match with the meal plan based on the usual intake. The results of your child's blood glucose tests will be used to fine-tune the match between food and insulin.

Table 2.1 shows how Lucy's (from Chapter 1) usual intake was translated into a carbohydrate counting meal plan. Notice, the dietitian didn't change Lucy's usual intake. She just translated Lucy's usual foods into carbohydrate gram equivalents to help with the insulin-balancing act.

Knowing what your child eats in terms of grams of carbohydrate, exchanges, or calorie points, etc., prepares you to adjust appropriately when variations in appetite or food availability inevitably occur. Depending on the situation and your own management approach, you might substitute another food, adjust an insulin dose, or encourage more or less activity to keep insulin doses in tune with the current situation. Each of these types of adjustments can be useful in keeping blood sugar control stable when life isn't.

CHECK FOR ADEQUATE FOOD INTAKE

There are two easy-to-check results that tell you whether your child is getting the right amount of food. One is a short-term test, and the other takes a longer view.

Hunger Is the Best Short-Term Measure of Adequate Intake

The short-term check is your child's level of hunger. If he's hungry all the time, chances are very good that he's just not getting enough to eat. If your child is constantly hungry, talk to your health-care team. Don't try to "tough it out" on your own. Withholding food from a hungry child is neither necessary nor helpful, and it's extremely hard on everyone. If it becomes a pattern, it can make the child desperate and obsessive about food. The meal plan, if your child has a set one, may need adjusting. Or the insulin plan might need improvement, so that your child can eat what is needed and get the food value from everything he eats.

Growth Is the Best Long-Term Measure of Adequate Intake

The long-term indicator of whether your child is eating the right amount of food is growth. Children grow normally only if they are getting the right amount of food. Your child's medical chart probably contains a growth grid, such as the ones shown in Figures 2.1 and 2.2 (infant charts are shown in

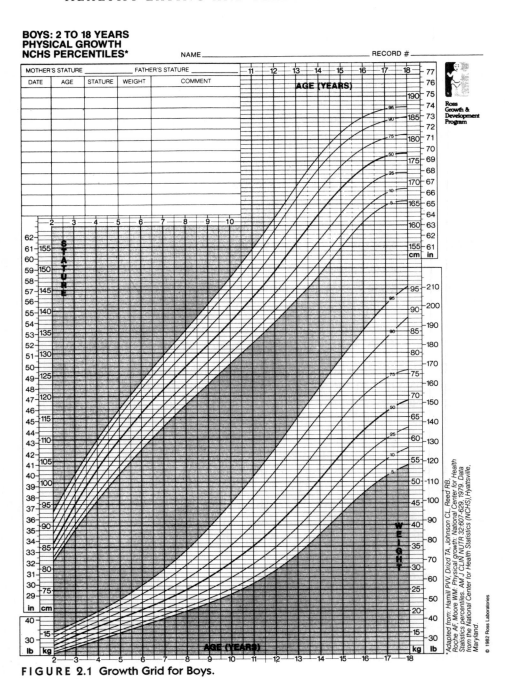

FIGURE 2.1 Growth Grid for Boys.

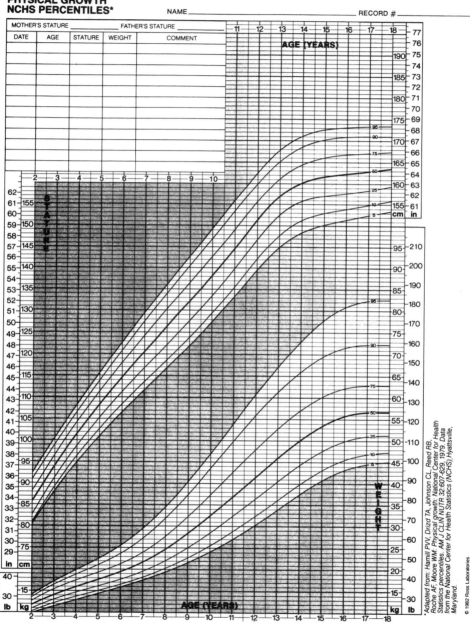

FIGURE 2.2 Growth Grid for Girls.

Chapter 10). These grids are based on the growth patterns of thousands of normally growing children. They allow you and your health-care team to track your child's pattern of changing height and weight in order to identify any changes from his usual pattern and to compare it to the average. You have a right to see and discuss the growth grid with your doctor or dietitian at your child's visits.

You'll notice that the grids have a series of curved lines already drawn in. Reading from the lowest line to the highest, the lines are labeled with the numbers 5, 10, and so on, through 95. These numbers are percentiles. The percentile number tells what percentage of the whole normally growing population of children at a given age were lighter or shorter than the number that falls on the line. The doctor, nurse, or dietitian enters your child's height and weight on the appropriate grid at each visit. In a medical version of "connect the dots," these values reveal a curved line that represents your child's unique growth pattern.

For example, the growth grid for 8-year-old Josh, whom you met in the **Introduction: What Diabetes Can Do to Families,** is shown in Figure 2.3. Josh's growth pattern for height had been around the 60th percentile since he was a baby. This means about 60% of kids were shorter than Josh at each age, and about 40% were taller. His growth slowed around the time his diabetes was diagnosed, because he was running out of insulin and couldn't grow properly. With treatment, things improved and his growth got back on track. However, his growth once again fell off his growth curve when his diabetes was in poor control and his meal plan was outgrown.

Notice that the grids include a space to fill in Mom's and Dad's stature (height). This gives the health-care team a reference point for judging whether a child is probably growing to his or her potential. Say Dad is a forward for the NBA and Mom can wash the top of the minivan without a step stool, but their 3-year-old's height is at the 15th percentile. The doctor or other health-care provider would watch that child's growth very carefully and check nutrition habits in detail, because the pattern would be unexpected in the child of

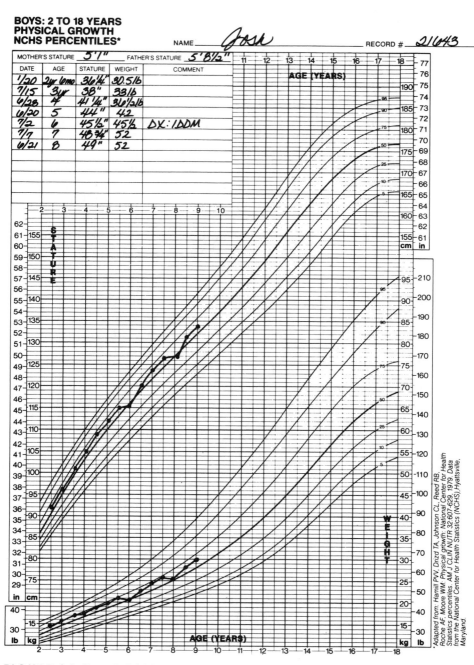

BOYS: 2 TO 18 YEARS
PHYSICAL GROWTH
NCHS PERCENTILES*

NAME _Josh_   RECORD # _21643_

MOTHER'S STATURE _5'7"_   FATHER'S STATURE _5'8½"_

DATE	AGE	STATURE	WEIGHT	COMMENT
1/20	2yr 6mo	36¼"	30.5 lb	
7/15	3 yr	38"	33 lb	
6/28	4	41¼"	36½ lb	
6/20	5	44"	42	
7/2	6	45½"	45½	DX: IDDM
7/7	7	48¾"	52	
6/21	8	49"	52	

*Adapted from: Hamill PVV, Drizd TA, Johnson CL, Reed RB, Roche AF, Moore WM. Physical growth: National Center for Health Statistics percentiles. AM J CLIN NUTR 32:607-629, 1979. Data from the National Center for Health Statistics (NCHS), Hyattsville, Maryland.

FIGURE 2.3 Growth Grid for Josh.

such tall parents. However, if Dad is a jockey and Mom sits on a pillow to see over the dashboard of the Mitsubishi, the 15th percentile would be seen as perfectly normal.

Keeping the diabetes in control by matching insulin to the right food intake allows a child to fulfill his or her genetic potential, which is most often similar to one or both parents. Occasionally, a child gets a blueprint like Uncle Mort (the only tall man in an otherwise short family) or Grandma Ellen (the only tiny, fine-boned person in a family of muscular, outdoorsy folks). If your child seems to be following a different pattern than the rest of the family, it may take awhile to figure out what his pattern is supposed to be. Each person's adult height and weight are reached according to a fairly predictable pattern of growth. That pattern can be followed from infancy through the teenage years using the growth grids.

Another important piece of information that can be obtained from the growth grid is a quick check of the relationship between height and weight. In spite of expectations created by the use of emaciated young girls to advertise everything from hiking boots to denture cream, people do come in different sizes and body types: thin, muscular, average, and heavy. For example, a girl with a muscular build might consistently follow a weight curve at the 70th percentile and a height at a somewhat lower percentile, say 60th. Or a boy with a slim build might consistently have a weight curve that hovers around the 50th percentile with a height curve a bit higher, perhaps at the 60th. Both the height and weight of a child with an average build would tend to fall at about the same percentile rank.

If there is a change in this established relationship, it's time for some detective work. For example, Julie had always been on the slim side, with a height around the 60th percentile and a weight around the 50th percentile. Over a 6-month period when she was 9 years old, her weight quickly moved up to the 65th percentile while her height stayed at around the 60th percentile. Even though Julie wasn't actually heavy, the pattern was unusual for her. It alerted her doctor to ask about an increase in hypoglycemia (and the extra food used to treat it) and to check her insulin doses.

In monitoring your child's growth, the important questions to ask the doctor, nurse, or dietitian are

- Do my child's percentile rankings for height and weight make sense for a member of our family?
- Is he or she staying on his or her own growth curve?
- Is the relationship between the height and weight percentiles appropriate and staying about the same?

If the answer to all of these questions is yes, then your child is eating the right amount of food for his or her own unique needs—even if he's eating a lot less than his brother did at the same age or he's eating twice as much as the other third graders. If the answer to any of these questions is no, his food intake, activity level, diabetes management, and general health need to be closely checked to see if there's a problem.

FOOD AND INSULIN BALANCE IS BASIC AND ESSENTIAL

The basic requirements for managing diabetes in kids are to 1) make sure they eat the right amount of food for their needs and then 2) give the right amount of insulin at the right time to allow their bodies to use the foods they eat. Although there are exceptions, most children with diabetes need about 3/10 to 4/10 of a unit of insulin for every pound of body weight (less during the temporary "honeymoon" that usually follows diagnosis, and up to twice as much during adolescence, when hormonal changes can increase insulin needs dramatically). For example, a 60-pound child will probably be on a total daily insulin dose of between about 18 units (60 lb. x 0.3 unit/lb.) and 24 units (60 lb. x 0.4 units/lb.) Keep in mind, however, that everyone is different. The best way to judge your child's insulin doses is how he's doing, not some average calculated number. Even if his dose is higher or lower than this average range, but he's

- Growing normally
- Active and energetic
- Not gaining or losing weight inappropriately
- Not routinely complaining of hunger

then both the amount of food being consumed and the total insulin dose are probably basically correct. Even though blood sugar control still may not be exactly where you want it to be, good growth and the absence of unusual hunger tell you that the big pieces of the care plan are in place.

On the other hand, if he has any of these problems:

- Growing poorly
- Gaining excess weight or losing weight unintentionally
- Having frequent low blood sugars
- Having frequent positive tests for urine ketones
- Experiencing generally poor glucose control

ask the health-care provider to review his insulin doses and food intake.

POOR DIABETES CONTROL CAN AFFECT APPETITE AND GROWTH

The indicators of adequate calorie intake—hunger and growth—apply to the child with diabetes, provided that the diabetes is in reasonable control. When blood sugar is running consistently high, however, the picture can get confusing. When the blood sugar level is fairly high (above 180 mg/dl for most people), sugar and all the calories it contains flow out in the urine. This can make it look like little George needs a lot more food than he is actually getting. It may seem he can "eat and eat and never gain an ounce." Or his growth may slow down because needed calories aren't staying in the body. If the child is getting too little insulin, his body will break down fat to get the energy it needs. When he's burning fat for energy, ketones will be produced and will show up in urine ketone tests. Ketones may lessen the child's appetite. Diabetes control needs to be improved before hunger will get back to normal and growth can proceed according to plan.

There is another diabetes-related situation that can make it tough to tell how much food a child really needs. This is when insulin doses are increased too much. Unfortunately, it's not all that rare for glucose levels to vary a lot during growth. Sometimes in our eagerness to control high blood sugars, we may increase the insulin too much, which then leads to low blood sugar. Although it doesn't happen often, it's easy to be fooled into "feeding" the extra insulin, instead of recognizing that too much insulin is being given. If this happens, the child may gain excess weight. To avoid these problems, insulin needs to be fitted to the child's food intake, not the other way around. That's one of the main reasons why it's so valuable for parents to learn how to make insulin adjustments.

We hope this gives you enough confidence to try out those parent and child job descriptions from Chapter 1. Remember, you get the right food into the house and on the table, and your child decides what he will eat of what's available.

THE BOTTOM LINE

In All Kids

1. Appetite is usually a good indicator of actual energy needs.
2. Energy needs depend on age, growth, size, and activity.
3. Hunger is the best short-term measure of correct calorie intake.
4. Growth is the best long-term measure of correct calorie intake.

In Children With Diabetes

1. Glucose control is required for normal growth.

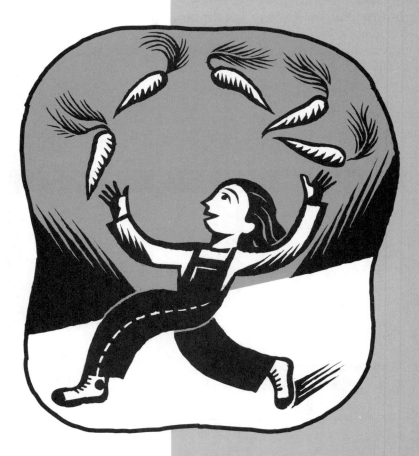

"Jody loves carrots, but giving her other vegetables is a waste..."

How to Tell if She's Eating the Right Things

Jody's mother was worried about the 4-year-old's rather limited menu of preferred foods. "There are so many things on the exchange lists that she should be eating, but she just doesn't like very many things. The only cooked vegetable she'll eat is carrots, and she actually gags when I give her broccoli. And what about bread? All she wants to eat is white bread or hamburger buns. Isn't she going to get sick if she doesn't start eating wheat bread pretty soon?"

When the dietitian learned a bit more about what Jody was eating, she was able to reassure her mother that the little girl was not in any immediate danger of developing malnutrition. Even though her preferred diet was pretty simple, even boring from an adult viewpoint, it was reasonably complete. People need certain nutrients, not certain foods, and Jody was getting enough of the right kinds of foods to provide the necessary nutrients.

Eventually her tastes expanded. She came to prefer the darker breads and a wide variety of the vegetables, salads, and dried beans that made up most of her parents' meals. But it took quite a bit of time, patience, and persistence before her tastes changed.

Mom and Dad just kept putting those things on the table and eating them themselves. They gave Jody lots of choices and frequent chances to try new things without pressure. The foods she liked were there for her to choose from, as well. At age 4, she simply preferred plain chicken or hamburger, cooked carrots, a few raw fruits and vegetables, white bread and buns, Cheerios, and milk. She ate those things with pleasure, but she was very suspicious of foods with coarser textures and stronger flavors.

People need certain nutrients, not certain foods, and Jody was getting enough of the right kinds of foods to provide the necessary nutrients.

● ● ● ●

It's perfectly fine for a youngster like Jody to eat virtually the same thing for dinner night after night, as long as the meal is nutritionally adequate and preparing it is not a burden. (If the diet is quite limited, a daily children's vitamin and mineral supplement may give you the reassurance you need until her tastes mature). Having preferred foods available increases the chances that the child will eat a normal-size meal. Trying to force hated or unfamiliar foods on a struggling child guarantees family food fights will occur, not to mention the fact that it violates your job description.

Still, Jody's mom was right to be concerned, because getting the right kinds of foods is very important. We all need the right raw materials to build and maintain a healthy body. This is equally true for every member of the family. The old saying "You can't make a silk purse out of a sow's ear" conveys the logical fact that you have to start with the right materials to make just about anything. You need silk, not pigskin, to make a silk purse. Likewise, you need protein, around 50 different vitamins and minerals, and a certain amount of energy to make healthy human bodies.

ONE HEALTHY DIET FOR ONE HEALTHY FAMILY

As far as we know, well-controlled diabetes does not change the body's need for calories, protein, or the vitamins, minerals, and other nutrients needed for health. The same foods that are best for everyone else in the family are also best for the child with diabetes. You will all feel and perform your best and have the best chances for long-lasting health if you eat a nutritious diet. Every family member will benefit from better nutrition, not just the child who has diabetes. On the other hand, uncontrolled diabetes, like many other stresses and environmental insults that we are all exposed to, may create a need for even more of the good things the body uses. One of the ways diabetes does this is by increasing the loss of some nutrients through the urine when high blood sugars cause a large volume of urine to be passed. All the more reason for the child with diabetes to be getting most of her diet from basic, nutrient-rich foods, along with the rest of the family.

Aside from the benefits to physical health, feeding everyone the same reasonable and healthful diet can help avoid many arguments, resentments, and feelings of being deprived. Basically, there is no easy way to feed your child with diabetes differently from the rest of the family. It certainly will create more work, and it will probably lead to hurt feelings, as well.

Still, every family is different, and you will need to weigh the pros and cons of the "one healthy diet for one healthy family" approach for your particular situation. The benefits include better health for everyone, reduced preparation demands (compared with preparing separate foods for family members with diabetes and those without), less pressure on the child with diabetes because there aren't so many "no's" in the house, fewer resentments from the child with diabetes because family members aren't eating forbidden fruit in her presence, and others that might be unique to your family. The most likely downside of this approach is resentment from other family members who may feel their freedom is being stepped on.

You, and you alone, can decide what works best for your family. Talk it over. Find out what everyone thinks and feels about any changes you are planning. See if you can come to an agreement about how to handle any concerns. The more changes that you're considering, the more important it is to talk it all out.

CHANGE FOOD PATTERNS GRADUALLY

If there is willingness to go ahead—with or without reservations and doubts—experiment with the new order. Say you'd like to try switching the whole family from whole milk to 1% milk. Consider taking a month to phase in the change (it takes time to adjust, so try to make all your experiments long enough to take this into account). Switch to 2% milk for at least 2 weeks. Then check out the level of adjustment before taking the step down to 1% milk. Other experiments in healthy eating might involve switching from chips to pretzels or from regular ice cream to a low-fat type, or not keeping big bags of chocolate kisses in the pantry for Dad's snacking. We strongly recommend this step-by-step approach, gradually taking away foods or making substitutions that the whole family can buy into. The same sort of approach can be helpful in adding more healthful foods to family menus. For example, it may take several tries to find vegetables that are a hit with everybody.

What if you have a family member who just won't give up certain foods? We've had more than one mom and dad who experimented with buying and eating their "guilt" foods late at night while the child with diabetes was sleeping, then disposing of the evidence before going to bed. Even though this has worked for some families, it's not an approach that we like to recommend. There's a real risk for fireworks and hurt feelings when and if your child discovers your empty Dove Bar wrapper in the trash one morning.

In the end, however, every family has to find its own way. Some have decided to keep certain junk foods around, working out a way for their child with diabetes to either avoid them or work them into her meal plan, often in smaller amounts than other family members. Your family's ultimate strategy will probably be a combination of eliminating some foods, limiting others, and substituting for still others until you have a healthier but probably not totally sin-free menu that incorporates every family member's wishes and needs to some extent.

Regardless of what foods are in the house or on the menu, it's certainly true that we need to keep track of how much and when the child with diabetes eats in order to manage the food, insulin, and exercise balancing act. But what is eaten can be the same for all family members, if you can work out the details.

HOW DID NUTRITION GET SO COMPLICATED?

Throughout most of human history (and in many nonindustrialized societies even today), there were very few decisions involved in eating. Tradition and simple availability determined what people ate. Today in the United States and other industrialized countries, however, choosing healthful foods can take a lot of thought and consideration. Guidelines and advice are everywhere. Why do we need to use our heads, instead of our appetites, in choosing what to eat? It is primarily because we now have a huge and rapidly expanding variety of foods to choose from, most of which are quite new.

For thousands of years, until quite recently in the big scheme of things, all the people of a given country, culture, or religion ate essentially the same foods. And all of those foods came from their own region, because the technology to transport and modify foods just didn't exist. Over a long period of time, the foodways of each culture evolved to include the right mix of foods from the local area that kept people healthy. Those who chose well were strong, powerful, and able to reproduce. People noticed what these healthy people ate and incorporated it into their own diets.

For example, even though no one even knew what calcium was until fairly recently, every traditional diet provided it. Peoples that kept cows or goats typically got their calcium from milk. But in most cultures, adults never drank milk, so other sources were found. For societies that ate ground grains, such as corn, the grinding stone usually added the needed calcium. People from fishing cultures ate calcium-rich fish bones. The same is true for all the essential nutrients. Iron comes from meat in some traditional diets, from leafy vegetables in others, and from blood and even cooking pots in still others. Asians get most of their protein from fish, pork, and eggs, while the major sources of protein in India are lentils, grains, and curd (yogurt).

Every traditional diet includes sources for all the essential nutrients. There was a simple, essential wisdom to grinding corn in a limestone metate if you grew up in Mexico or to eating raw liver after a big hunting kill if you were a Bushman. Living the modern life, however, we don't do those traditional things anymore. Now, with nothing but our taste buds and ability to pay to guide us, we can make some pretty awful choices. The incredible increase in obesity and the rising tide of heart disease and other chronic conditions make the result of those poor choices very clear.

In addition to the disappearance of traditional foodways and the appearance of many new foods of doubtful nutritional value, we also are challenged by the easy availability of food. Before the mass production and transportation of food became common, food was not easy to come by. You had to hunt it, grow it, or gather it from the countryside. Then you had to skin it, clean it, chop it, and cook it from scratch to make it edible. All of those things were hard work. They took much more effort than driving to the corner market and loading up a shopping basket or, for an even more dramatic change, faxing your shopping list to a grocery store that delivers. Surpluses were carefully preserved for later needs (more hard work) and then eaten a bit at a time, not wiped out in one Saturday night food orgy.

Our situation today is very different. Fast-food restaurants seem to be on every street corner. Pizza is only as far away as your phone. Huge bags of chips lie in the pantry, ready for a little light grazing at the end of the day. And triple fudge ripple ice cream fills the freezer and calls your name, even when you're not hungry. It's all so easy, and it tastes so good! Most of us can get literally anything we want at a fairly reasonable cost. Between easy access and the powerful influence of advertising hype, most people in the United States today eat an extremely wide variety of foods, not all of which have much of a track record for supporting human health.

Very few people eat the time-tested traditional foods of their ancestors. Even when they do, it's most often special celebration and holiday foods, not the common, everyday selections that guaranteed good nutrition. For example, most baked goods and sweets take a long time to prepare. When they had to be made at home, they showed up on the table infrequently, mostly at special occasions. Now they're available every day at low cost. Someone else has done all the work, making them so much more available that they are likely to displace more essential foods.

The problem then, in a nutshell, is that we have lots of choices, too many of those possible choices are nutritionally poor, and we no longer follow time-tested traditional food patterns. How can we choose well under the circumstances? After all, you need to be able to make good choices. It's vital to the health of the whole family. It's the information you need to fulfill the first part of the parents' job description: *get the right stuff on the table.*

A SIMPLE GUIDE TO GOOD NUTRITION

Thankfully, there's an uncomplicated tool you can use to plan nutritious meals for the whole family. It's called the Food Guide Pyramid. You've probably seen it on cereal boxes and loaves of bread many times. The American Diabetes Association and The American Dietetic Association adapted the Food Guide Pyramid into a Diabetes Food Pyramid.

The Diabetes Food Pyramid, shown in Figure 3.1, divides foods into six groups, because no one food contains all the

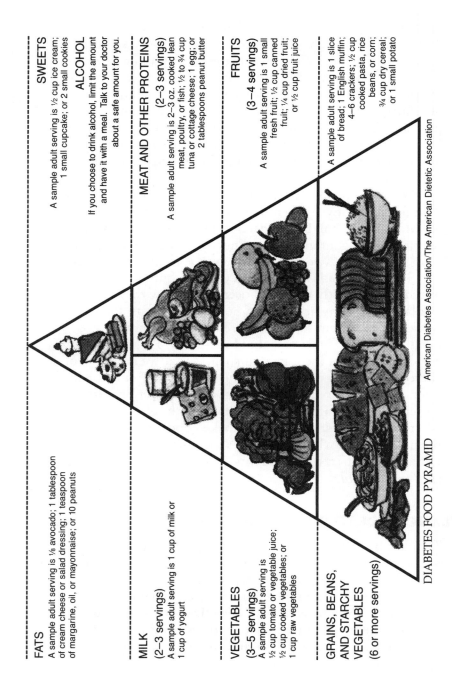

FATS

A sample adult serving is ⅙ avocado; 1 tablespoon of cream cheese or salad dressing; 1 teaspoon of margarine, oil, or mayonnaise; or 10 peanuts

SWEETS

A sample adult serving is ½ cup ice cream; 1 small cupcake; or 2 small cookies

ALCOHOL

If you choose to drink alcohol, limit the amount and have it with a meal. Talk to your doctor about a safe amount for you.

**MILK
(2–3 servings)**

A sample adult serving is 1 cup of milk or 1 cup of yogurt

**MEAT AND OTHER PROTEINS
(2–3 servings)**

A sample adult serving is 2–3 oz. cooked lean meat, poultry, or fish; ½ to ¾ cup tuna or cottage cheese; 1 egg; or 2 tablespoons peanut butter

**VEGETABLES
(3–5 servings)**

A sample adult serving is ½ cup tomato or vegetable juice; ½ cup cooked vegetables; or 1 cup raw vegetables

**FRUITS
(3–4 servings)**

A sample adult serving is 1 small fresh fruit; ½ cup canned fruit; ¼ cup dried fruit; or ½ cup fruit juice

**GRAINS, BEANS, AND STARCHY VEGETABLES
(6 or more servings)**

A sample adult serving is 1 slice of bread; 1 English muffin; 4–6 crackers; ½ cup cooked pasta, rice beans, or corn; ¾ cup dry cereal; or 1 small potato

DIABETES FOOD PYRAMID

American Diabetes Association/The American Dietetic Association

FIGURE 3.1

TABLE 3.1 Minimal Daily Nutrition Requirements: Portion Sizes Change With Age

Food Group	Infant	Toddler & Preschooler	School Age	Teen
Milk	16–24 oz.	2 cups (no more than 3 cups)	2–3 cups	4 cups
Breads/ Cereals	4 servings, about 1–2 tbs. or 1/4 the adult serving each	4 servings, about 1 tbs. per year of age or 1/4 the adult serving each	4 adult or exchange size servings	4 adult or exchange size servings
Fruits/ Vegetables	4–5 servings, 1–2 tbs. or 1/4 the adult serving each	4–5 servings, about 1 tbs. per year of age or 1/4 the adult serving each	4–5 adult or exchange size servings	4–5 adult or exchange size servings
Meat/ Protein	2 ~1/2 oz. portions	2–3 oz.	2–3 oz.	4–5 oz.

needed nutrients.[1] However, given nutrients are consistently found in certain kinds of foods. For example, calcium is found in all dairy products, and vitamin C is found in fruits and vegetables. If we eat from all the right groups every day, we get what we need without being tied down to eating certain foods that we may not like or that may not be available.

The Pyramid shows the types of food and the relative amount of each type of food that we need to eat each day. The Pyramid shows the minimum number of adult servings needed for adequate nutrition. Table 3.1 shows how serving sizes change with age, as a child's size and needs change.

- *Grains, beans, and starchy vegetables* make up the largest portion of the Pyramid, just like they should make up the largest portion of the overall intake. They are the base or the backbone of a healthy eating plan and should be a major source of energy (calories). They provide essential B vitamins and iron, and, if you

---

[1] Human milk is an exception to this "no perfect food" rule, and it's only adequate for infants.

choose whole-grain varieties, they also are a good
source of fiber and trace minerals, like chromium and
copper.

- *Fruits and vegetables* make up the next largest block of
  the Pyramid. They are important sources of several
  vitamins, especially vitamins A and C, and many
  minerals, including trace elements. Make at least one
  choice high in vitamin A (like carrots, dried apricots,
  cantaloupe, dark greens, or sweet potatoes) and
  another high in vitamin C (like broccoli, oranges,
  peppers, cabbage, or strawberries).
- *Dairy products* make up part of the next level of the
  Pyramid. They are an important source of calcium,
  protein, and vitamin D. Low-fat varieties are the best
  choice for fluid milk products, yogurts, and cheeses,
  once a child is past the toddler stage.
- *Meat and other proteins* make up the other part of the
  third Pyramid tier. Depending on the type of protein
  food chosen, they are important sources of iron and
  other minerals, as well as some vitamins.
- *Sweets and fats* are shown in the tiny top portion of
  the Pyramid. These foods provide extra calories and
  enjoyment once basic needs are met, but if eaten in
  large amounts, they can keep us from eating the
  things we really need. Fats include those added in
  cooking or at the table. Eating according to the
  Pyramid means limiting sweets, fried foods, gravies,
  sauces, margarine, and salad dressings to modest
  levels.

Eating the minimum number of servings each day from
the Pyramid gives kids the minimum amounts of protein,
vitamins, and minerals their bodies require. Of course, most
children need to eat more than that minimum number of
servings in order to get the amount of energy (calories) that
their growing bodies and level of physical activity demand.
It's like the bank requiring you to keep $500 in your checking
account to avoid penalty charges, but you actually need to

keep closer to $1,500 to pay your bills. For older, bigger, and more active kids who need more food, the remaining calories should come from the same groups and in the same general proportions shown on the Pyramid. Meet kids' excess energy needs by offering more or bigger portions of the basic food groups. Keep the relative proportion of fats and sweets small, compared with the amounts of starches, fruits, vegetables, proteins, and dairy foods. This will pay off in better short-term well-being and better long-term health than meeting all that excess energy demand with nutritionally poor foods like sweets and high-fat snacks. This is just as true for Mom, Dad, and the rest of the kids as it is for the child with diabetes.

A NOTE ABOUT VEGETARIAN DIETS

Vegetarian diets seem to be much more common than they once were. There are several approaches to vegetarian eating. Some people avoid only red meat. Others avoid all types of animal flesh. Another type of vegetarian avoids animal products altogether, including milk, cheese, and eggs. Not only are there different types of vegetarian diets, there are also many different reasons why people adopt a vegetarian eating style. For some, it is a requirement of their religion. For others, it is a response to concerns about the environment. Others avoid meat because of an ethical aversion to killing animals. Still others find a vegetarian eating style either economical or more healthful. Some people with diabetes are drawn to a vegetarian diet because some research suggests that vegetable protein is easier on the kidneys than animal protein. Whatever the belief or reason behind it, eating a vegetarian diet is perfectly compatible with both good health and good diabetes control. Vegetarians, too, can use the Diabetes Food Pyramid as a nutritional blueprint. It's just that the foods in the Protein section will include cheese, eggs, beans, peas, lentils, tofu, soy products, etc., rather than meats. Total vegetarians (or vegans), those who avoid all animal products, would not use cheese or eggs, and for them, the

Dairy or Milk group will consist of soy milk rather than cow's milk products.

A couple of cautions are in order, however. Total vegetarian diets—that is, those with no animal products at all—can be hard for very young children to digest. If this happens, they may have problems getting enough calories and protein. Vegetarian diets are much more bulky than diets that include meat, cheese, and milk. To help overcome this problem, it is probably best to include at least milk and eggs as protein sources in the diets of kids of preschool age and younger, and to make sure adequate fat is added in cooking and at the table to provide enough calories in the small volume of food that these very young children can eat. It is also important to make sure that hard-to-digest foods—beans and cracked grains, for example—are cooked thoroughly and then mashed or chopped to help along those young jaws and intestinal tracts. As for all youngsters, especially those with diabetes, monitor the growth of very young vegetarian kids. Appropriate growth is the best indication that they're getting all the nutrients and energy they need.

Another caution relates to a couple of nutrients that are more of a challenge to get in vegetarian diets: iron and vitamin B_{12}. Most nutritionists and doctors recommend supplements of these nutrients for kids and adults who are eating vegetarian diets.

The final point regarding vegetarian diets is directed specifically at your child with diabetes. It is not a problem, just a difference in management that you need to be aware of. Meat, fish, and poultry don't affect blood sugar very much. Neither do some of the vegetarian sources of protein, such as eggs, peanut butter, tofu, and cheese. Some vegetarian protein foods, however, contain considerable amounts of carbohydrate that need to be counted when matching food and insulin. Beans, lentils, and black-eyed peas, for example, have quite a bit of carbohydrate. In fact, we included them with starches on the Diabetes Food Pyramid to make it easier to remember to count their carbohydrate value. If your child with diabetes is

TABLE 3.2 What Two Real Kids Eat in a Day

Pyramid Group	Lindy, 4 years old	Jason, 10 years old
Grains, Beans, and Starchy Vegetables	3/4 cup cereal, 1 slice sandwich bread, 5 pretzels, 11 miniature graham bear cookies, 1/2 of a dinner roll	1 1/2 cups cereal, 4 slices sandwich bread, 15 pretzels, 25 miniature graham bear cookies, 1 baked potato, 2 dinner rolls, pizza crust from 1 slice
Fruits	1/2 cup apple juice, 1 fresh apricot, 1/2 cup strawberries	8 oz. apple juice, 2 apricots, 1 cup strawberries, 1 banana, 1 kiwifruit
Vegetables	3 carrot sticks, 1/2 cup green salad, 4 cherry tomatoes	6 carrot and celery sticks, 1 1/2 cups green salad, 4 cherry tomatoes, 2 stalks steamed broccoli, 1 can vegetable juice
Milk and Dairy Products	2 cups milk	2 cups 2% milk, 1 carton low-fat yogurt, 1 cup chocolate milk
Meat and Other Proteins	1 slice cheese, 1 slice roast beef	3 oz. string cheese, 3 tbs. peanut butter, 3 slices roast beef, 1 slice cheese pizza
Sweets and Fats	1 tsp. mayonnaise, 1 tsp. salad dressing, 1 tsp. margarine, 5 gummi bears	2 tsp. mayonnaise, 2 tbs. salad dressing, 3 tsp. margarine, 2 oz. lite sour cream, 10 gummi bears

following a vegetarian eating style, don't forget to count the carbohydrate value of the high-starch protein foods it's likely to include.

HOW WHAT REAL KIDS EAT FITS INTO THE PYRAMID

Table 3.2 shows what a normally picky 4-year-old girl and her active 10-year-old brother each ate in one day. Both are eating according to the Pyramid, but the amounts are very different because Lindy and Jason differ in age, size, and activity level.

Can you tell from looking at the foods listed in Table 3.2 which of these children has diabetes? Both children are eating from all the Pyramid groups, and both are eating small amounts of sweets in keeping with the Pyramid pattern. It's Jason who has diabetes. Lindy, like Jody whom you met at the beginning of the chapter, has pretty simple tastes, but all the types of food required for good health are there.

IS THIS NORMAL PICKINESS OR IS MY CHILD ABNORMAL?

What about children who have truly odd food preferences? Or unusual eating behaviors? How can you tell (and what can you do) if your child's food choices seem to be abnormal? Normal eating varies—a lot! In fact, it varies so much that we've been having a hard time coming up with a simple definition to put down here for you. Every time we think we've found a reasonable guideline, we think of all the exceptions to the rule. From the first time a baby is put to the breast, a unique eating personality is apparent. Food preferences, speed of eating, even the noises kids make while they eat, are individual. That's what makes it hard to draw a clear line between normal and abnormal eating.

Some kids seem to have unique or unusual taste preferences. Most babies and young children seem to prefer milder flavors and neutral or sweet foods over things that are sour or bitter. But beyond these normal characteristics of younger palates, some kids are just "wired" for greater taste sensitivity. Remember, every adult wine taster and gourmet cook started life as a kid—probably one who drove his mom crazy. Keep in mind that you can't taste what your child is tasting. Their own immature taste buds, inexperienced palate, or personal degree of flavor or odor sensitivity may give them a very different experience of any given food than what you are having.

But be patient. Nothing is set in stone. Foods that were once accepted willingly or even demanded can suddenly end up on the 10 Most Hated List (and vice versa, too.) Think of foods you once hated but eventually learned to enjoy. If you can remember how your own tastes have changed, it may help you deal with your child's current food preferences.

On the personality side of picky behavior, some people are just suspicious of anything new and are slow to make changes. The first reaction to any new food for kids with this type of personality will probably be to resist eating it. Other children are very open to new experiences of all kinds, and food is just part of that general outlook on life. You know your own child. The way she responds to food will probably just be an extension of her overall approach to life. You won't change it. The child will probably change somewhat with age and experience, but whether she does or not, keep your cool. Keep mealtimes pleasant to ensure that food is not a source of arguments. Food fights are a losing battle in any family. But they're especially harmful in the family facing diabetes.

There is no food that everybody *has to like. And nobody has to like* everything.

• • • •

When they balk at foods, remember your job description. Get a variety of the right kinds of foods on the table and eat them yourself. Set your own mealtime rules and enforce them. Maybe in your house, everybody has to at least taste everything that you serve. Maybe you're training your kids to quietly say, "Thanks, Mom, but I don't care for anymore," instead of tossing a half-chewed morsel on the table and shouting, "Yuck, that's gross!" Whatever your rules are, be consistent.

As far as knowing when a quirky eating preference or behavior may actually be a cause for concern, consider the following points:

- Remember that there is no food that *everybody* has to like and eat. And nobody has to like *everything*. It's natural to want to eat more of the foods we like and less (or none!) of the foods we dislike. As long as your child is eating some choices from all the food groups of the Pyramid, she'll do fine nutritionally. As for the terminally picky, they will probably be all right in the short run if they eat some choices from each level of the Pyramid (for example, a child who refuses all vegetables but eats fruit, or a child who won't eat meat but takes dairy products). But if your child's choices stay that limited for more than a few weeks, we'd recommend having a dietitian do a nutritional analysis of several days of the child's intake. This is the best way to find out if this behavior is putting her at any real risk. Observe your child's growth, general health, and energy level. If they're good, then chances are excellent that her insisting on having a peanut butter sandwich for lunch every day is not causing any serious problems. Food jags will almost always die a natural death if you don't make a big deal out of them.

- Does your child seem to enjoy her food? If so, this is a good sign that no major problems with food exist. On the other hand, if she's tense and seems overly worried about either having or avoiding certain foods, it might be a good idea to consult with a physician, dietitian, or counselor.

- If anything about your child's eating drives you so nuts that you can't let it slide, get some help in evaluating it. There really may be an eating problem, or you just may need some help in better dealing with your child's normal quirkiness. Either way, a pediatric dietitian or a family counselor will probably be able to help. See Chapter 9 for more about preventing, identifying, and, if necessary, treating seriously disordered eating.

You can use the Diabetes Food Pyramid to plan nutritious meals for the whole family. Healthy eating won't eliminate enjoyment, favorite foods, or special occasions. Every food fits into the Pyramid somewhere, because every food can be a part of a nutritious eating plan. Every food also can fit into a diabetes meal plan, but more about this in Chapter 5. Variety is important. Offer it, but relax. Children will build up their repertoire of preferred foods slowly over time. You can support this process through your own healthful eating, especially if you don't pressure your child to eat certain foods. By questioning and experimenting, you can develop a way of dealing with food that will promote good health for the whole family. That same plan can work for your child with diabetes, reducing or even eliminating many of the food-related stresses that have troubled you in the past. For more information on the Food Pyramids, see the resource list at the end of Chapter 4.

THE BOTTOM LINE

1. People need certain nutrients, not certain foods, to be healthy.
2. All foods can be included in a healthy eating plan for the child with diabetes as well as other family members.
3. Withholding sweets makes them seem more desirable than other foods. Plan them into meals in appropriate amounts so they can be enjoyed without displacing needed nutrients.
4. The Diabetes Food Pyramid can be the basis of both healthful family meals and the diabetes meal plan.
5. Some kids are picky, but likes and dislikes change with age and experience.
6. Keep getting the right stuff on the table, and kids will eventually learn to like most of it.

II SECTION

• • • • • • • •

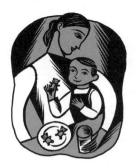

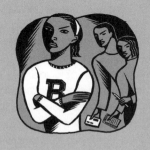

The second section covers issues that are unique to diabetes. We describe lots of food and insulin management techniques that will make it possible to balance diabetes management needs with parenting needs when conflicts arise.

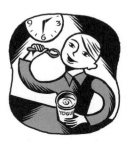

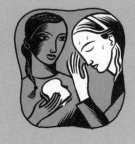

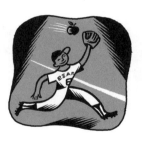

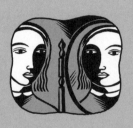

Nutrition and Meal Planning in Diabetes

The second section covers issues that are unique to diabetes. We describe lots of food and insulin management techniques that will make it possible to balance diabetes management needs with parenting needs when conflicts arise. We discuss how to best help the obese or thin child whose appetite doesn't appear to be working as it should. We suggest ways to promote desirable food choices and ways to deal with poor choices when they happen.

In Chapter 4, we describe how food affects blood sugar and how you can use that information to best coordinate your child's food intake with insulin and exercise. We also talk about how sweets are handled to keep blood sugar under control. We describe how to minimize, prevent, or deal with the blood sugar changes that might be caused by variations in appetite. We talk about ways to handle the diabetes fallout from actions like asking the child to leave the table in the middle of a meal if she's misbehaving.

In Chapter 5, we introduce you to the process of setting blood sugar goals and cooperatively solving problems as a family. To be successful, you will need to apply what we offer to your own unique family situation. You also may need to rethink some of your ideas about child rearing. If you're able to stretch in these ways, we think you'll be really happy with the results.

In Chapter 6, we describe the role of snacks in the overall nutrition of young children. We detail the special value of snacks for children with diabetes, describing how they provide protection against high and low blood sugars. We offer an approach for using snacks to better manage variations in children's appetites.

Chapter 7 is intended to help you cope more effectively with low blood sugar. We begin by describing the many symptoms of low blood sugar, so you'll know what you are looking for. Then we talk about the common causes of hypoglycemia and discuss its consequences. Finally, we offer practical suggestions for increasing your and your child's ability to recognize, avoid, and treat low blood sugar.

In Chapter 8, we describe the many benefits and the few, but important, risks that exercise holds for a child with diabetes. We discuss the best ways we've discovered for reducing those risks. There is also some specialized advice geared to very young kids, to youngsters who are into organized sports, and to less active children. And specifics on how to make those food and insulin adjustments to prevent hypoglycemia during exercise are included.

In Chapter 9, we discuss eating problems and clinical eating disorders, from the merely frustrating to the truly dangerous. As we discuss each type of problem, we tell you its signs and symptoms, its causes and consequences, and offer hints for preventing and dealing with it.

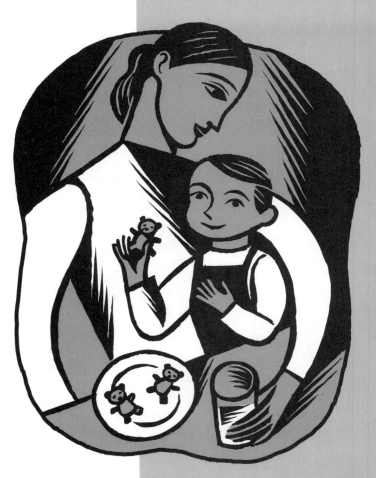

"I know I would be totally demoralized by someone doling out
11 Teddy Grahams to me, and I won't do it to José ..."

The Basics of Diabetes Nutrition and Meal Planning

José's mother is to diabetes strategy what General Patton was to the 7th Army in World War II: a mover and a shaker.

José's mother, Ann, is more than a mere survivor of the battle to help her child live well with diabetes. She is even more than a warrior. She is to diabetes strategy and chutzpah what General George Patton was to the 7th Army in World War II: a mover and a shaker. Ann has worked very effectively to keep her family's life and meals as normal as possible. Her thoughts about living with José's diabetes mirror those of many parents with whom we've worked.

"As soon as diabetes entered the picture, food took on a larger-than-life role. It would have been so easy to lose all the joy of preparing and eating food, because we had to constantly think of things that were never an issue before: timing of meals, for instance, and the ingredients in everything. Food is a very personal thing, and a lot more than nutrition goes into choosing what we eat. But diabetes can take you to the point where it seems like all you're thinking about are the hard facts: how big a portion? how much carbohydrate?

"The way diabetes dominates family meals can make it seem like you've lost a basic freedom. And the 'foreverness' of diabetes can be overwhelming, too. That's why I feel it's so important not to overdo the rigid diet attitude. Nobody can stay rigid all the time."

We couldn't agree more. Our work with so many families over the years has convinced us that overly rigid guidelines — "Eat exactly this, no more and no less," "Never let your child eat that"—are unrealistic, unproductive, and, most importantly, unnecessary. We believe strongly that the more you know about nutrition, diabetes, and effective family problem-solving, the more freedom you will have. Real freedom. With knowledge, practice, and problem-solving, you can earn an impressive degree of freedom in food choices, greater meal-timing options, and the enjoyment of family meals free of food fights. Notice that we said "earn," because these gifts don't just waltz in off the street. You work for them. But we think they're more than worth the effort.

THE BASICS OF NUTRITION AND DIABETES

Why is food such an important part of every plan to manage diabetes? Because diabetes takes away the body's ability to properly use the energy from foods. And since energy is essential for life and health, restoring that ability is the major focus of treatment.

The food we eat breaks down into a form of sugar called glucose. Glucose is the body's main fuel—like gasoline is the fuel that runs your car. When the glucose from digested food enters the bloodstream, the bodies of people who don't have diabetes release insulin so that sugar can enter body cells. Once in the cells, glucose is used to keep the heart beating, the muscles moving, etc.

Because your child's insulin-producing cells don't work anymore, that system can't do its job. Without effective management, insulin is not where it's supposed to be when it's supposed to be there. Bingo! Glucose builds up in the bloodstream instead of going to cells, so the body is starved for energy. In addition, tissues get damaged because glucose is flooding a lot of places in the body where it's not supposed to be.

Before he had diabetes, your child's pancreas automatically and precisely produced and released the insulin his body needed. It put in more insulin when he ate. It put in less when he was active. It met whatever his needs were, exactly. Now that automatic system no longer works and you're in the business of "playing pancreas." Working from the outside, you and your child try to balance food, insulin, and exercise, using the results of blood glucose testing to guide you. Since food is the major thing that determines insulin needs, you need to know what was eaten and how much insulin it takes to handle it in order to keep the diabetes under control. When you pull off that balancing act successfully, the blood sugar level hovers somewhere near the normal range.

A BASIC CHANGE IN HOW WE THINK ABOUT DIABETES MEAL PLANNING

Nearly all health-care providers used to believe that someone with diabetes should control everything about their lives—especially food and exercise—to match the prescribed insulin doses. Those doses were seldom changed, and when they were, it was done only by the doctor. This approach put good blood sugar control out of the reach of everyone but the most rigidly disciplined people. Perhaps worse, it created tremendous stress and restrictions for everybody else. Because of improvements in our treatment tools—especially because of the availability of home blood glucose monitoring—that old, rigid approach is becoming much less common, especially among health-care providers who specialize in diabetes.

Today, most diabetes specialists prefer physiological therapy. This means that we now try to come closer to what the body did before diabetes developed. We try to match injected insulin to the individual situation, instead of trying to cram your child's life into a box created by an average insulin dose or standard schedule of shots. This change in thinking not only has made better control possible for more people with diabetes but also has greatly reduced the amount of stress and restriction needed to achieve that control. The old diabetes therapy was often unsuccessful, at least partly because it didn't leave room for human nature. Constant self-control and discipline were needed to achieve reasonable diabetes control using urine testing and less physiological insulin regimens. As Ann pointed out at the beginning of the chapter, nobody can stay rigid all the time. The updated diabetes therapy uses new and better tools to make diabetes care much more realistic and user-friendly.

Our new approach to food is a very clear example of this change in thinking. "One size fits all" diabetes meal plans are no longer accepted as adequate. Instead, it is now considered best to base each person's diabetes meal plan on his usual eating habits, and then design the insulin regimen to fit that situation. In Chapter 2, we describe how the plan is developed, using a good record of what and when a child usually eats. The plan may be somewhat different from what the child was eating previously. For example, food may be moved around to create a pattern that provides better protection against low blood sugars. Or, amounts may be varied if a child is significantly above or below a desirable weight range. But as many as possible of the previous eating habits are incorporated into the diabetes meal plan.

For most people, insulin doses now change more frequently than they did in the past, perhaps even daily. In addition, the changes are often made by the individual with diabetes or his family rather than by the doctor or other health-care provider. These more frequent changes can greatly improve blood sugar control. They can also provide greater flexibility—freedom to eat a wider variety of foods, to eat different amounts on different days, to sleep in occasionally, to do all sorts of spur-of-the-moment things—without losing blood sugar control.

Does this mean that your child can now forget about following a diabetic diet? That he can eat whatever he wants, whenever he wants? Yes and no. From the standpoint of general nutrition, the rules are the same for the child with diabetes as they are for everyone else. If he ate junk all the time, his health would suffer, even if you and he could manage to control his blood sugar while he did it. But since virtually any food can be included in a healthful eating plan, he can eat anything he wants to, as long as it's done so that needed foods aren't excluded. From the perspective of blood sugar control, as well, it is possible for your child to eat anything he wants. But to do that and maintain good diabetes control requires quite a bit of work. "Playing pancreas" is a demanding job. It requires keeping track of what's eaten and then learning the specific effect of that food on blood sugar and insulin needs. How much insulin does it take to balance Grandma's special chocolate birthday cake? Do they even make enough insulin to handle a large deep-dish pepperoni pizza? The answers to such questions will be unique for your child. But you can find them, just like you can find workable ways to deal with everyday meals. The process starts by understanding, in general, how different foods affect blood sugar.

THE EFFECT OF FOODS ON BLOOD SUGAR AND INSULIN NEEDS

All foods, except pure alcohol, add sugar to the bloodstream, but not in equal amounts. Around 90 to 100 percent of carbohydrates (starches and sugars) enter the bloodstream as glucose. Much less protein and fat are broken down into glucose. In addition, the glucose from carbohydrates tends to show up in the bloodstream shortly after eating, while the glucose from proteins and fats tends to appear in the blood up to several hours later. The amount of insulin needed to control blood sugar after meals depends mostly on the amount of carbohydrate eaten. The most basic fact about diabetes meal planning is that you need to know how much carbohydrate your child eats in order to keep food and insulin in balance.

WHERE'S THE CARBOHYDRATE?

Carbohydrates are found in varying amounts in

- Fruits and vegetables, and the juices made from them
- Grain products, such as breads, rice, cereal, and pasta

- Starchy vegetables, such as potatoes, sweet potatoes, and corn
- Dried or canned beans, peas, and lentils
- Dairy products, particularly milk and yogurt
- Sugar-sweetened foods, such as cake, candy, pie, cookies, ice cream, and regular soda.

All of these foods can be part of a healthy diet (but in different proportions, as described in the previous section on the Diabetes Food Pyramid). All of these foods add sugar to the bloodstream. All of these foods need to be balanced by insulin and/or exercise, or they will drive the blood sugar far above the normal range. Various tools can help you with this task.

DIABETES MEAL PLANNING TOOLS

The most common diabetes meal planning tools are the food exchange and carbohydrate counting systems. They both work. So do less common systems, such as calorie points and total available glucose (TAG), among others. Personally, we think that carbohydrate counting gives you and your child more flexibility in food choices and is a bit easier to learn than the other approaches. But you may already know the exchanges. Or your dietitian or other health-care provider may prefer some other system entirely. That's fine.

The exact system you use is not really important. What is important is using the basic concept of balancing insulin with the carbohydrate content of what's eaten and knowing how to use your own system well enough to include all the foods that are important to your family.

The Diabetes Food Pyramid, which we described earlier as a guideline for healthy eating, can be your bridge between family meals and diabetes meal planning. Look at the Diabetes Food Pyramid in Figure 4.1. It shows how the Pyramid relates to food exchanges and carbohydrate counting. Notice how the sections of the Pyramid correspond to the food exchange groups and how a carbohydrate value can be assigned to servings from each Pyramid group. If you use the Diabetes Food Pyramid to plan meals for the whole family, you can

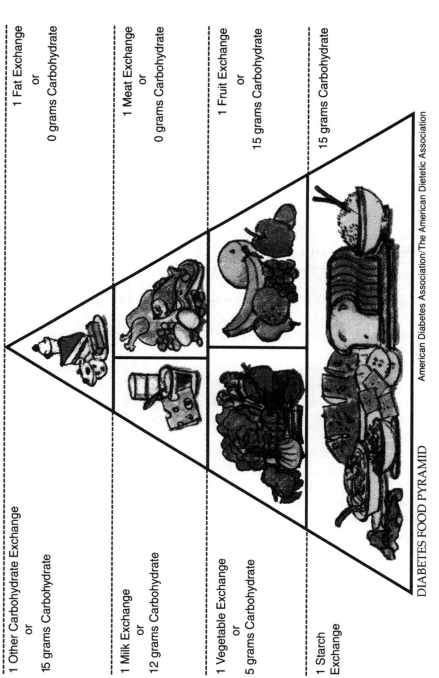

1 Fat Exchange
or
0 grams Carbohydrate

1 Other Carbohydrate Exchange
or
15 grams Carbohydrate

1 Meat Exchange
or
0 grams Carbohydrate

1 Milk Exchange
or
12 grams Carbohydrate

1 Fruit Exchange
or
15 grams Carbohydrate

1 Vegetable Exchange
or
5 grams Carbohydrate

15 grams Carbohydrate

1 Starch
Exchange

DIABETES FOOD PYRAMID

American Diabetes Association/The American Dietetic Association

FIGURE 4.1

TABLE 4.1 Food Groups of the Exchange System

	Carbohydrate g	Protein g	Fat g	Calories
Carbohydrate Group				
Starch	15	3	1 or less	80
Fruit	15	0	0	60
Milk	12	8	0–8	90–150
Other Carbohydrates	15	varies	varies	varies
Vegetables	5	2	0	25
Meat and Meat Substitutes Group	0	7	0–8	35–100
Fat Group	0	0	5	45

keep track of what your child with diabetes eats within that same Pyramid structure.

With food exchanges, the meal plan is made up of a given number of servings from each of three major food groups: Carbohydrate, Meat and Meat Substitutes, and Fat. Table 4.1 shows how foods are divided into groups in the food exchange system and the average nutrient content of a serving from each group.

Because it describes everything eaten, an exchange meal plan covers both general nutrition needs and diabetes control in a single tool. In a major move toward greater flexibility, the 1995 revised version of the exchange system (the one shown here) encourages people to exchange among all the carbohydrate-containing food groups. A lot of people say they find the exchange system confusing. This probably relates to the fact that many people don't get enough instruction in exchanges to use them effectively. Several nondiabetes meal planning approaches—including Weight Watchers and Deal-A-Meal—have been based on this versatile meal planning tool.

In carbohydrate counting, the meal plan consists of a target number of grams of carbohydrate for each meal and snack or a number of 15-gram carbohydrate servings. Any combination of foods and serving sizes that provides the given amount of carbohydrate can be chosen. Food labels, exchange lists, food composition books, or a combination of these sources can provide the needed information.

Table 4.2 illustrates how a food record is viewed in terms of the Diabetes Food Pyramid, the food exchange system, and

TABLE 4.2 Expressing Jody's Usual Intake in Different Systems

Jody's Food Record	Pyramid	Exchanges	Carb Counting
Breakfast			
1/2 cup Cheerios	1 Bread/Grain	1/2 Carb (Bread)	7 g
1/3 cup 2% milk	1/3 Milk/Dairy	1/3 Carb (Milk)	4 g
1/4 banana	1 Fruit	1/2 Carb (Fruit)	7 g
3 oz. orange juice	1 Fruit	1 Carb (Fruit)	12 g
			Meal Total = 30 g
Morning Snack			
1 slice white toast	1 Bread/Grain	1 Carb (Bread)	16 g
2 tbs. peanut butter	1 Meat/Protein	1 Meat/Substitute	0 g
1/3 cup 2% milk	1/3 Milk/Dairy	1/3 Carb (Milk)	4 g
			Meal Total = 20 g
Lunch			
1 oz. hamburger patty on	1 Meat/Protein	1 Meat/Substitute	0 g
1/2 hamburger bun	1 Bread/Grain	1 Carb (Bread)	15 g
6 carrot and celery sticks	1 Vegetable	1 Carb (Vegetable)	5 g
1/3 cup milk	1/3 Milk/Dairy	1/3 Carb (Milk)	4 g
1 oatmeal raisin cookie	1 Bread/Grain	1 Carb (Bread)	11 g
			Meal Total = 35 g
Afternoon Snack			
1 soft pretzel stick with	1 Bread/Grain	1/2 Carb (Bread)	6 g
1 oz. soft cheese	1 Meat/Protein	1 Meat/Substitute	0 g
1/2 cup apple juice	1 Fruit	1 Carb (Fruit)	15 g
			Meal Total =~20 g
Dinner			
2 oz. baked chicken	1 Meat/Protein	2 Meat/Substitute	0 g
1/2 cup cooked carrots	1 Vegetable	1 Carb (Vegetable)	8 g
1/3 cup mashed potatoes	1 Bread/Grain	1 Carb (Bread)	12 g
1/2 cup vanilla pudding with	1 Sweet/Fat	1 Carb (Other) + 1 Fat	17 g
1 pineapple ring	1 Fruit	1/2 Carb (Fruit)	7 g
1/2 cup 2% milk	1/2 Milk/Dairy	1/2 Carb (Milk)	6 g
			Meal Total = 50 g
Bedtime Snack			
1 oz. sliced chicken on	1 Meat/Protein	1 Meat/Substitute	0 g
1 slice white bread	1 Bread/Grain	1 Carb (Bread)	15 g
1/3 cup milk	1/3 Milk/Dairy	1/3 Carb (Milk)	4 g
			Meal Total =~20 g

carbohydrate counting. The record shown is an average or composite day for Jody, the 4-year-old you met in Chapter 3. This was Jody's usual intake at the time, and it was used to design her basic diabetes meal plan.

SOURCES OF MEAL PLANNING INFORMATION

No matter what meal planning system you and your team choose, you'll need information about the nutritional makeup of the foods your family eats. You'll use that information to fit those foods into your child's meal plan. Chances are, your team will provide you with some tools to get you started: an exchange food booklet or a list of the carbohydrate grams in certain foods.

Don't think that just because a food isn't included in the literature that came from your dietitian, it can't be part of your child's menu. The world is absolutely chock-full of different kinds of foods, and they can all be worked into a diabetes meal plan if you have the right information. It's possible to have an extremely varied diet and still maintain diabetes control. Knowledge is power. Knowledge about the nutrient contents of the foods your child wants to eat will allow you to go for the gusto!

The best source of that information is the Nutrition Facts label on packaged foods. The content of the label is dictated by federal regulations, and you can rely on its accuracy. Most packaged and processed foods have one of these labels that lists the amounts of calories, carbohydrate, protein, and fat in a specified serving of the food, as well as other information. Figure 4.2 shows a sample Nutrition Facts label for a low-fat granola bar.

The information you'll be using most will be the calorie, carbohydrate, fat, and protein values. Depending on the meal planning system you're using, you may need one, two, or even all of those values to figure out how the food fits. If you're counting grams of carbohydrate, you can take the value directly off the label. If you're counting carbohydrate exchanges or servings, divide the Total Carbohydrate value on the label by 15 to get the number of "carbs" provided by a serving of the food. If you're using one of the other meal planning systems, ask your dietitian or other health-care provider how to convert nutrition label information into the measure used in your particular system. Regardless of the meal planning approach you're using, be sure to check the serving

Nutrition Facts

Serving Size 1 bar

Servings per Container 10

Amount per Serving

Calories 110 **Calories from Fat** 20

	% Daily Value
Total Fat 2g	3%
Saturated Fat 0.5g	3%
Cholesterol 0mg	0%
Sodium 100mg	4%
Total Carbohydrate 22g	7%
Dietary Fiber 1g	4%
Sugars 10g	
Protein 2g	

FIGURE 4.2

size shown on the label against the amount your child actually eats: is it more, less, or the same? If necessary, adjust the nutrient values to the actual portion eaten.

Reliable food composition information can also be found in brochures from several national restaurant and fast-food chains. If, after trying all these sources, you need even more information, consider investing in a good book on food composition. Some are listed in the recommended reading list at the end of the chapter.

BLOOD GLUCOSE MONITORING RESULTS TELL THE TALE

The right basic meal plan and insulin doses are important, but they're only a starting point. To reach your goals for control, for family lifestyle, and for flexibility, you need to respond every day to a changing situation. Blood glucose changes from hour to hour and day to day. Physical activity increases and decreases. Food intake varies a little or a lot. And many other things—some that we understand and some that we don't—subtly or radically change the diabetes control game on an almost daily basis. To keep up with the ever-changing show, you need a certain amount of timely information to allow you and your child to respond appropriately. There's no other way to keep blood glucose in control. That's the real process of making diabetes management work. And it depends absolutely on regular blood glucose monitoring. There is no other source of information that is as necessary or as powerful.

How much testing you'll do depends on blood glucose goals, insulin regimen, financial issues, and your child's acceptance of the routines, among other things. Your diabetes team can help you work out the best plan for your particular situation. Most kids require a minimum of four tests (before meals and at bedtime) to achieve control throughout the day. Occasional tests at around 3 A.M. are used to check for overnight lows, and more frequent tests are needed during illness and exercise. Some teams also use after-meal tests to check out the match in doses and timing between food and insulin.

However many tests you, your child, and your team agree upon, make sure you're getting all the benefit possible from every single finger stick. First of all, make sure those numbers don't get lost. You or your child may write them down or you may be relying on meter memory. But being able to look at them in relation to each other and to insulin doses and food intake is absolutely vital. If you're new to this process, you'll be looking at all that information with your dietitian, nurse, doctor, or other team member. Later, you'll do it on your own. You'll be looking for patterns: patterns that are related to certain days of the week, certain activities, or certain types of meals. You'll start with a basic skill, such as following a written plan for adjusting insulin doses according to how much carbohydrate is being eaten. With practice, you may become able to take multiple factors into account—not only food, but also current blood glucose, activity that came before, activity that will come after, and so on. But that level of skill only comes with lots of practice.

To get maximum benefit from blood glucose testing, you also need to be clear about what the goals are for various times during the day and what to do about specific values. For example, a blood glucose of 100 mg/dl is probably within your target range for a before-meal reading: no action is needed other than, perhaps, breathing a small prayer of thanks to the cosmos! But a reading of 100 mg/dl at bedtime may be another story entirely. It may be lower than what your team has determined is safe to go to bed on. What should you do? Change the bedtime snack? Probably. But how, exactly? Having a specific action plan is vital. Otherwise, testing can be extremely frustrating. The motivation to test quickly fades when people don't know what to do about the results. That's one of the many reasons that it's so important to keep working with your team. They can transfer knowledge and skill to you in a step-by-step fashion, just as you can ultimately transfer it to your child.

But before you try out for the Diabetes Management Olympics, it's necessary to examine the match between your child's basic meal plan and his insulin doses.

GETTING INSULIN ADJUSTED TO A BASIC MEAL PLAN

We assume that you eventually want to learn to adjust insulin for variations in food intake. But to get there you have to "pay your dues" by following a less flexible approach. You'll need to spend some time—at least a couple of weeks, but probably longer—sticking as closely as possible to your child's basic meal plan. Consistently eating the same amount of carbohydrate at each meal and snack makes it much easier to use blood sugar test results to fine-tune insulin doses and timing. The more food intake varies during this period, the longer it will take to figure out the precise relationship between food and insulin. As you know, however, consistency is not always easy to come by. Children have variable appetites from day to day, and we have made quite a point of how inadvisable it is to force or withhold food when the child's appetite disagrees with the meal plan. However, if the child is old enough to understand and cooperate, some simple adjustments can make it easier to keep carbohydrate intake stable, in spite of variations in appetite. These techniques can take some of the sting out of a set meal plan during the important stage when insulin/food relationships are being worked out. These same techniques are also very helpful in everyday management for families who are just not ready to start adjusting insulin on their own yet.

WAYS TO STICK BY A MEAL PLAN WHEN APPETITE VARIES

When the child is still hungry after eating the planned meal, foods with little or no carbohydrate can be added without affecting the blood glucose level. Try foods like celery and other raw vegetables, diet gelatin, meat, cheese, peanuts, and seeds. For example, if Jody was still hungry at lunchtime after eating her usual half a sandwich, vegetable sticks, milk, and cookie (see Table 4.2), her mom could give her the choice of peanut butter on celery sticks, a slice of cheese, or a handful of peanuts. None of these foods is likely to raise Jody's blood sugar very much, but they would satisfy her hunger in a way that was acceptable to her.

If, on the other hand, Jody was not feeling hungry enough to eat all of the usual meal, her mom could use one or both of the following techniques. She could give priority to the carbohydrate-containing foods, perhaps removing some of the meat or vegetables from the table when she saw that Jody wasn't as hungry as usual. She could also give the carbohydrates in a more concentrated form so Jody would get all the needed carbohydrate in a smaller package. For example, she could substitute half a cup of fruit juice for the milk and cookie or for the slice of bread.

CHOICES PAVE THE ROAD TO CONSISTENCY

Helping your child with diabetes to eat the actual amount of food (grams of carbohydrate, number of exchanges, calorie points, etc.) planned is an important part of daily diabetes management. This is somewhat less of an issue if you are adjusting insulin. After all, the decision about how much will be eaten is made only about 30 minutes before the meal, when the insulin dose is taken. The child won't change his mind by the time he sits down to eat. Right? Hah! It still happens. And, of course, if you are trying to follow a specified meal plan to which your child's set insulin doses have been matched, the struggle comes up even more frequently. The child is either ravenous or uninterested. He either hates what you're having for dinner or wants to eat the whole casserole because he loves it so much. Given what we've said about the problems associated with either forcing or withholding food, what's the answer?

Parents tell us the answer is choices. By offering a variety of choices that are all acceptable, you get out of the "eat it or else" business. Instead of having only one carbohydrate choice on the table, routinely offer two or three and make at least one of them something you know your kid will always eat. Many families we've worked with have some staple offerings that are always in the fridge or on the table. Milk, apple sauce, canned peaches, white bread, instant mashed potatoes, creamed corn, and fruit yogurt are often on the list for younger children. Older youngsters may have more exotic preferences. When a child is given choices instead of ultimatums, the chances of his getting balky and refusing to eat shrink dramatically.

Likewise, always offer some choices that don't raise blood sugar much, so your child can have more to eat if he's still hungry without throwing diabetes control into a cocked hat. Some possibilities are second helpings of the meat or other protein, vegetables with dip, green salad, nuts, and other low-carbohydrate foods. If the amounts of protein added to a meal are quite large, you may find a rise in blood sugar some hours after the meal. A portion of protein can be converted to glucose under certain circumstances. We describe later how to take advantage of protein's delayed effect on blood glucose by including some in bedtime snacks.

If your child frequently wants much more or less than is on the meal plan, the plan may need adjusting. Talk to your dietitian or other diabetes educator.

HOW DO SWEETS FIT INTO A DIABETES MEAL PLAN?

The carbohydrate in sweets needs to be part of your meal or snack total. Both the exchange and carbohydrate counting systems make it easy to do this. We think one of the best ways to handle the actual offering of sweets is to set out the dessert right at the beginning of the meal with everything else. We like this method because it avoids making sweets into something so special that you have to eat all the healthier foods to get them. (It's a valuable approach for any other children in the family as well as for the child with diabetes.) This positions sweets appropriately for good nutrition as well as for diabetes control. They become just another part of a healthy diet—something we enjoy in modest amounts without guilt. In terms of diabetes management, it conveys clearly that all carbohydrate foods are equally important to blood sugar control.

HOW IMPORTANT ARE PORTION SIZES?

Portion sizes are quite important. After all, knowing how much carbohydrate is eaten is what makes it possible to keep insulin well-matched to your child's needs. Anybody who's "playing pancreas" needs that information. How precise you need to be, however, is another one of those things that's unique to your child. Generally, the smaller the body size, the more important it is to be precise. A given amount of carbohydrate, say 15 grams, will raise blood sugar a whole lot more in a 40-pound body than it will in a 120-pound body. But body weight is not the only factor. Kids of the same weight can have different responses to the same amount of carbohydrate, just like they might have quite different total insulin doses. We sometimes think that the only thing that's the same about all kids with diabetes is that they're different! Experience will show you whether you need to be exact with your child's portions to get the control you're after, or whether rough estimates will get the job done.

Regardless of whether you're counting every gram of carbohydrate or generally estimating exchange-size servings, ideally, controlling portions will not be tied to *limiting* what your child eats as much as it will be to *knowing* how much carbohydrate he takes in. Remember that the best indicator of how much your child needs to eat is nearly always his appetite. Neither forcing nor withholding food works in the long run. But to keep food and insulin in sync, you and he really need to know how much carbohydrate he eats. Can you accomplish this without being the old ogre that counts out exactly 11 Teddy Grahams to a waiting child? We think so.

One of the best ways to handle sweets is to set out the dessert right at the beginning of the meal with everything else.

● ● ● ●

Doling out just so much to a hungry kid is not fun. This is especially true if the rest of the family is diving in like a pack of hungry wolves. The quote from José's mom, Ann, that starts this chapter expresses the bind that many parents feel in being the gatekeeper for serving sizes. It isn't a problem in all families, but if it is in yours, here are some things that may make things easier. See how they work with your family.

One option is to serve up everyone's plates before bringing them to the table, restaurant-style. Another is to portion foods before cooking, as in making individual casseroles. You can also portion out foods into dishes that control the serving size; for example, always filling the cereal bowl or the fruit bowl to the same level. This is a reasonable way to handle the 11 Teddy Grahams dilemma. Maybe there's a small plate or bowl that the little cookies can be shaken into that holds your child's standard portion. What if the amount that your child wants to eat or that fits in the serving dish isn't the same as the serving size for which you have information? Figure it out. Say the little dessert plate actually holds about 16 or 17 Teddy Grahams. (Pour a portion out two or three times, count or measure each one, and then take the average.) Use simple multiples or fractions of the value you know. If 11 Teddy Grahams equals one Starch Exchange or 14 grams of carbohydrate, count your little dessert plate serving as 1 1/2 Starches or 21 grams of carbohydrate.

Prepackaged portions can also be helpful. Try individually wrapped granola bars (instead of a whole plate full of cookies), single cups of yogurt, or individually wrapped ice cream bars (instead of serving out of a gallon container). Those prepackaged portions are nearly always well labeled so you know exactly how much carbohydrate they contain. Whether you will be serving up food at the table or in the kitchen, look for serving spoons that dish out a known amount. A serving spoon that accurately dishes out half a cup is particularly useful because so many carbohydrate foods have a standard serving size (for which you know or can learn a carbohydrate value) of 1/2 cup. That same 1/2-cup serving spoon can also be used to estimate other sizes of servings (a scant spoon full is 1/3 cup, a half a spoonful is 1/4 cup, two spoonfuls is a cup, and so on). Use as many of these simple techniques as you find useful to make servings consistent. If your serving sizes are consistent, even if they're not exactly half a cup or whatever, you'll get the insulin adjusted to the consistent serving over time. The amount normally portioned out becomes a habit. Kids learn the portions by osmosis.

Some people bite the bullet for a time and weigh and measure portions so that their eyes get trained. If you're going to do this, you'll need measuring cups and spoons. And if you're using a system that includes controlling meat portions, you may also want to use a portion scale to weigh those for a while. Keep in mind, though, that many people who have gone through this training process tell us their eyes get untrained over time. Portion sizes tend to slowly grow until they are nowhere near the intended serving. Therefore, it's helpful for those who estimate portions by eye to occasionally go back to measuring, to keep their eyes properly calibrated. Some families actually go on weighing and measuring forever because they are precise about everything. The trick is to find methods that are comfortable for your family and lifestyle. It's our impression that families who are consistently successful find ways to integrate portion control right into their food serving and preparation techniques.

SOME FINER POINTS OF CONTROL

Timing Meals and Insulin

Excellent blood sugar control is most likely when insulin is matched in both amount and timing with the sugar from digested food. Even if the correct amount of insulin is taken, the blood sugar level can still rise too high right after the meal if the insulin is taken too close to mealtime. On the other hand, if your child is an incredibly slow eater, his blood sugar may actually fall too low while he's eating, because the insulin has arrived in the bloodstream before enough food has been eaten to balance its effect. The traditional way to manage this is to closely dictate the amount of time before eating that the insulin should be taken. Thirty to 45 minutes is a pretty standard recommendation for those who take Regular (R), NPH (N), or Lente (L) insulin. The very best delay is an individual thing that can be worked out by paying attention to after-meal blood sugar results. For example, if blood sugars are too high right after a meal but come down into the target range before the next meal, we know the dose is correct, but the timing could use improvement. One solution is to plan more time between the shot and the meal. But as we've already mentioned, many people have a very hard time waiting to eat.

Luckily, there is another technique that works quite well. The body digests and releases glucose from different kinds of food at different speeds. We can use that information to improve the match between insulin and food.

Carbohydrates tend to release sugar into the bloodstream fairly quickly, creating an immediate need for insulin. Protein and fat have a much slower and less strong effect on blood sugar. We can delay insulin demand (when Regular, NPH, or Lente insulins are taken too close to the meal) by leaving the carbohydrate foods alone until the end of the meal. Start with salad. Then serve the meat and vegetables. Leave the bread, potato, fruit, and other high-carbohydrate foods until last. Dividing the food up in this way pushes the biggest need for insulin out farther after the meal, closer to when the insulin will peak.

What about the child who eats incredibly slowly or the situation where insulin was taken and then dinner got delayed for some reason? In these cases, the carbohydrate foods can be eaten first, rushing sugar into the bloodstream to cover the peaking insulin. Meat, salad, and vegetables can be eaten last. In short, there are several ways the insulin-meal interval can be adjusted to fit a kid's style. Very fast eaters may do fine with a short delay between the shot and the meal, especially if the carbohydrate is loaded toward the end of the meal. A short delay may also be best for a child going through a period where his appetite is very poor or unpredictable, and he eats slowly. Giving insulin 30 minutes before the meal in this kind of situation can end up giving everyone ulcers. Mom and Dad can get so anxious for the child to eat that trying to hurry him along is all but unavoidable. In this situation, insulin could be given very close to the meal or even afterward. Neither of these is a perfect solution, but they can help preserve the child's safety while also protecting family relationships.

Adjusting Insulin Doses for Altered Food Intake

There is a relationship between the grams of carbohydrate your child eats and the amount of insulin his body needs to use them. That ratio can be used to calculate the appropriate bolus (premeal dose of Regular insulin) for any meal or snack. The carbohydrate-to-insulin ratio varies quite a bit from person to person. Most children need about one unit of insulin for every 15 to 20 grams of carbohydrate. In general, the lower the total daily insulin dose, the greater the amount of carbohydrate covered by one unit of insulin. To find your child's unique value, start with an estimate and test it. Some people start with one unit for every 15 grams of carbohydrate, since this is the value of a Carbohydrate Exchange serving and it makes calculations simpler.

1. Test your child's blood glucose value before eating. It should be in his target range. If it's too high or too low, the actual effect of the insulin dose (premeal bolus) being tested will be unclear.

2. Plan a meal of known carbohydrate content. This could be his usual meal according to his basic meal plan, or it could be a test meal, such as 1 oz. of cereal, 8 oz. of skim milk, and 4 oz. of juice (equals 45 grams of carbohydrate).

3. Calculate the bolus for the test meal using your estimated ratio. For example, 10-year-old Guy plans to eat the 45-gram carbohydrate test meal described above. He's using an estimated sensitivity factor of one unit for every 15 grams of carbohydrate. The dose being tested is three units of Regular insulin.

4. Test blood glucose after the meal, and adjust the ratio as needed. The blood test can be done from 2 to 5 hours after the meal. If, for example, you want to keep your child's 2-hour after-meal blood sugar values below 180 mg/dl, you might want to do the test 2 hours after the meal. Or, if your goal is to have your child's blood sugars between 90 and 140 mg/dl before meals, you may want to just test before the next meal. If the reading is higher than the target value after the test meal, then try a lower insulin-to-carbohydrate ratio (more insulin per amount of carbohydrate) at the next meal. For example, if Guy consistently had a 2-hour postmeal blood glucose of more than 200 mg/dl with the three-unit bolus, he might try using one unit of insulin for each 10 or 12 grams (instead of 15). On the other hand, if the after-meal blood sugar was below the target range or he had a hypoglycemic reaction, he would need to adjust the ratio so that he was getting less insulin for the same amount of carbohydrate, perhaps one unit for every 17 or 20 grams. He would continue testing and adjusting until his glucose targets were achieved.

Once you and your child have figured out this relationship, the correct insulin dose for any meal can be found easily, whether your child is very hungry, wants to indulge in an unusual special occasion meal, or doesn't feel very hungry at all. Now that's flexibility!

Insulin and Meal Adjustments for Out-of-Range Blood Sugars

Modifying meal-related insulin doses according to what's being eaten works best when the blood sugar at the beginning of the meal is in your child's target range. But, of course, that's not always the case. Blood sugar is very often higher or lower than it's supposed to be. To get the best possible blood sugar control, it's necessary to respond to the out-of-range reading. There are various approaches that can be of help.

One of the best tools for responding to out-of-range blood sugars is a specific system (sometimes called an algorithm or sliding scale) for adjusting insulin based on the current blood sugar level, usually the value obtained at mealtime. High blood sugar means there's too little insulin around. In addition to whatever insulin will be needed to cover the meal, extra insulin will be required to correct that high blood sugar. Low blood sugar means there's been too much insulin around. Some of the extra can count toward the needs for the coming meal, meaning less insulin can be given.

Some people guesstimate what those adjustments should be, giving one to two units more or less than the usual dose. Some people don't make these kinds of adjustments at all. They may not know how, or they may have had a bad experience adjusting in the past. We feel, however, that these adjustments are appropriate and helpful for most children with diabetes. For most people to be successful with insulin adjustments, they need a more rational and consistent approach than guesstimating. That's why we advise using an individualized insulin adjustment factor to make this kind of dose change. Your doctor or educator may have helped you work one out already. If not, we have a simple way to identify one that should be fairly accurate for your child. It's called the 1,500 Rule.

Developed by Dr. Paul Davidson, an endocrinologist from Atlanta, Georgia, this rule says to divide the number 1,500 by the total daily insulin dose. The resulting value is the number of mg/dl that one unit of Regular insulin will lower the blood sugar. (We'll skip the rather complicated explanation of why this works and just tell you that 1,500 is a constant that Dr. Davidson identified in working with his very large group of people with diabetes.)

For example, the total of all of 12-year-old Andy's insulin doses (all the Regular plus all the NPH) is 30 units. According to the 1,500 Rule, we would expect one unit of Regular insulin to reduce Andy's blood sugar by about 50 mg/dl. Andy and his parents use that value to tweak his insulin doses before meals, taking into account the blood sugar test result. Say his blood sugar before the evening meal is 264 mg/dl, but his goal is to have his blood sugars between 90 and 120 mg/dl before meals. He'll need some extra insulin to correct that high blood sugar, provided he's planning to eat his usual dinner. Using his adjustment factor of one unit of Regular for every 50 mg/dl of blood sugar, his parents calculate that he should add three units to his premeal dose. The extra three units should bring his blood sugar back to about 114 mg/dl. That would allow the meal-related insulin dose to really do its job. Otherwise, the blood sugar is likely to be just as high or higher after the meal as it was before. If Andy wasn't feeling hungry enough to eat all of his usual dinner (some children have reduced appetite when blood sugar is high), the need to increase the dose would be less. See Table 4.3 for another example of how to calculate an insulin adjustment when blood glucose is above the target range.

The same calculation, using the 1,500 Rule, can be used to reduce the premeal insulin dose if the blood sugar is too low before the meal. If Andy's blood sugar was only 60 mg/dl before dinner, his usual premeal dose could be reduced by a unit to help correct the low. However, if Andy was extra hungry because of his low blood sugar before the meal, he might just want to eat more. This would remove the need to lower the insulin dose.

Some doctors advise waiting for the premeal insulin to bring high blood sugar down nearer to the target range before

TABLE 4.3 Calculating a High Blood Sugar Insulin Adjustment Factor Using the 1,500 Rule

Lisa is 8 years old. She takes 17 units of insulin a day (3 1/2 units of Ultralente [U] and 4 units of Regular [R] before breakfast, 3 units of R before lunch, and 3 1/2 units of U and 3 units of R before dinner).

Calculating Lisa's Insulin Adjustment Factor:

1,500 ÷ 17 = 88 mg/dl (drop in blood glucose for each unit of R insulin).

Situation: Lisa's blood glucose
before supper is   252 mg/dl
           − 120 mg/dl (highest blood glucose goal before meals)
           = 132 mg/dl (difference ÷ 88 = 1 1/2 units of R insulin adjustment).

Solution: Add 1 1/2 units of R to Lisa's usual 3-unit predinner dose to correct the high blood glucose.
Adjusted dose = 4 1/2 units of R and 3 1/2 units of U.

starting the meal. This is a really hard sell with a hungry child. You can get some of the same effect without having to delay the meal by following our earlier suggestion of first feeding the child things that don't raise the blood sugar (salad, vegetables, meat). Leave the carbohydrate foods until the end of the meal, when the insulin has had some time to start working on that high blood sugar.

Making insulin and food adjustments is a skill that you and your child can develop through trial, error, and a lot of practice. Your doctor or educator may be a good resource to help you trouble-shoot any difficulties that come up when you first use this approach.

If making insulin adjustments is not comfortable for your family, your other option for responding to out-of-whack blood sugars is to modify the food intake. This may not be as satisfactory as making an insulin adjustment, especially if your child really wants to eat more or less than the planned amount. Trying to withhold food when blood sugars are high is likely to create battles. In fact, when parents try to routinely hold back food because of high blood glucose, kids may become reluctant to be honest about high numbers. On the other hand, you probably won't encounter much resistance giving extra food to a child whose sugar is running low before a meal.

The third option is to adjust the basic dose of insulin, based on a pattern of high or low blood sugars, instead of, or in addition to, adjusting the immediate dose each time you get an out-of-range reading. Say Andy needed to add two or three units of extra insulin at dinnertime for 3 days in a row because of a high blood sugar value. On the 4th day, he could add two or three units to the basic dose of the insulin responsible for the reading at that time of day. In his case, it would be his morning dose of NPH. For another child, it might be a prelunch dose of Regular. This approach is sometimes called a pattern-based insulin adjustment. Its purpose is to fix a pattern of out-of-range blood sugars.

Making insulin and food adjustments is a skill that you and your child can develop through trial, error, and a lot of practice.

• • • •

Regardless of which method or methods you and your child use, it's important to find comfortable, workable ways to respond to daily blood sugar readings. This is an important key to better blood sugar control. It also gives you a lot more return on the time, discomfort, and money you invest in blood sugar testing than just gathering up the numbers in a book for the doctor or nurse to review every 3 months or so.

Your child's meal plan for diabetes management is based on the same healthful eating selections that are best for the whole family. It's necessary, however, to have a system for figuring out how much carbohydrate he's getting from what he eats in order to keep his food and insulin in balance. All sources of carbohydrate affect the blood sugar—from brown bread to white sugar—and all need to be accounted for. It used to be assumed that people with diabetes had to control their eating to match their insulin doses. It's now much more common to adjust insulin to keep pace with a person's intake. Good nutrition is still a high priority, but we now have much more flexibility in how we achieve it.

RECOMMENDED READING AND RESOURCES

Food Pyramids

Diabetes Meal Planning Made Easy: How to Put the Food Pyramid to Work for You, by Hope Warshaw, MMSc, RD, CDE. American Diabetes Association, Alexandria, VA (1996).

The First Step in Diabetes Meal Planning. American Diabetes Association/The American Dietetic Association, Alexandria, VA (1995).

The Food Guide Pyramid. United States Department of Agriculture, Human Nutrition Information Service, U.S. Government Printing Office, Washington, D.C. (1992).

CSPI's Healthy Eating Pyramid. Center for Science in the Public Interest, Washington, D.C.

Exchange Meal Planning

Exchange Lists for Meal Planning. American Diabetes Association/The American Dietetic Association, Alexandria, VA (1995).

Exchanges for All Occasions, by Marion Franz, RD, MS. Park Nicollet HealthSource, Minneapolis, MN (1994).

Carbohydrate Counting

Carbohydrate Gram Counting: How to Zero in on Good Control, by Betty Brackenridge, Linda Fredrickson, and Chip Reed. MiniMed Technologies, Sylmar, CA (1995).

Getting Started (introduces concepts), *Moving On* (introduces pattern reading), and *Using Carbohydrate/Insulin Ratios* (adjusting insulin for changes in food or activity). American Diabetes Association, Alexandria, VA (1996).

Food Composition

Bowes and Church's Food Values of Portions Commonly Used, by Jean A.T. Pennington, PhD, RD. 16th edition. J.B. Lippincott Co., Philadelphia, PA (1994).

The Complete Book of Food Counts, by Corrinne Netzer. 3rd edition. Dell Publishing, New York NY (1994).

Fast Food Facts, by Marion Franz. 4th edition. Park Nicollet HealthSource, Minneapolis, MN (1994).

THE BOTTOM LINE

1. Food intake is inseparable from glucose control.
2. To ensure both control and growth, insulin doses should be matched to calorie needs, not the other way around.
3. The diabetes meal plan should be built on each child's usual intake.
4. Carbohydrates—starches and sugars—are the main source of blood glucose.
5. Keep track of all carbohydrates so that insulin can be kept in balance with intake.
6. Offering lots of appropriate choices promotes consistency without making Mom and Dad into "food police."
7. Learn to adjust insulin for changes in food intake to obtain the most flexibility and best control.
8. Learn to adjust insulin for out-of-range blood sugars using the 1,500 Rule or guidelines from your health-care provider.

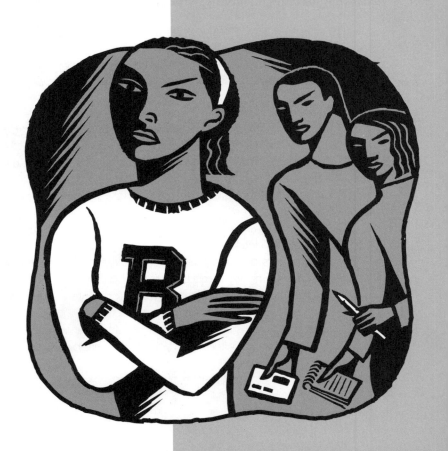

"The doctor wants Meghan's blood sugars to be perfect all the time..."

Beyond Blood Sugar Control: Diabetes Goals for Families

I'm worrying about her diabetes all the time now because she never does.

At 15, Meghan was having a hard time: a hard time with her diabetes, a hard time with her doctor, and a really hard time with her very frustrated parents. The pursuit of perfect blood sugar control was at the center of the storm. An advocate of good control, Meghan's doctor had always examined her blood sugar records very closely at every visit. She circled every number above 160 or below 70 mg/dl and then asked for an explanation of what had gone wrong. With a lot of hard work and dedication from both of Meghan's parents, this approach had consistently produced HbA_{1c} values of less than 8% since her diagnosis at the age of 7. (The HbA_{1c} test, also known as the glycosylated hemoglobin or glycohemoglobin test, measures average blood sugar control over the past 2 to 4 months according to how much sugar clings to red blood cells. The higher the blood sugar, the more "candy coating" on the cells.) Unfortunately, things had started to change about the time that Meghan turned 13 and had been getting steadily worse ever since.

The first sign of a change had been more variability in her home blood sugar test readings—higher highs, lower lows, and more of both. Then her HbA_{1c}s started to climb. This triggered lots of questions from both the doctor and her parents. They accused Meghan of not following her meal plan or of not taking her insulin when she was away from home. Soon, Meghan started "forgetting" to do her blood tests. When Mom or Dad forced her to do a blood test and the result was a high reading, it nearly always led to a big fight. By the time we saw them, Meghan was meeting her parents' frequent questions with stony silence.

"She doesn't follow a meal plan at all anymore," her father said. "She has an after-school job now, and I think she spends most of the money she makes eating at fast-food places with her friends. I keep telling her she's going to get complications, but she doesn't care. She just wants to do things with her friends. I'm worrying about her diabetes all the time now because she never does."

Meghan's parents' worry and frustration were absolutely understandable. All parents want their children to be healthy. But what does healthy really mean when your child has diabetes? It means good blood sugar control, of course. But it means much more, as well. It means being happy and self-confident, at least most of the time. It means that your child enjoys her friends, that she cares about things, and that she works hard at the things she cares about. That's the ideal; the reality is often dramatically less glowing. All too often, you may feel that the blood sugar part of your child's health is on a collision course with all the other parts, and that the big pileup is always just ahead. This is a problem every parent of a child with diabetes faces constantly. Isn't there some way out of this fix? Isn't there a way to help your child be healthy in every way? It might be hard to believe, but the answer is yes.

HOW IMPORTANT IS GOOD BLOOD SUGAR CONTROL?

Let's get one thing clear at the start. Good blood sugar control is important. For one thing, it has immediate benefits. Most children feel awful when their blood sugars are bouncing around. Low blood sugar (hypoglycemia) is always uncomfortable. It also can be embarrassing, scary, or even dangerous. Some children also feel rotten when their blood sugars are too high (hyperglycemia), but it's interesting that children are less likely than adults to say they feel bad at high blood sugar levels. Adults often feel exhausted and cranky when their sugar levels are high, while many kids say they feel fine or even have more energy. If your child feels fine when her sugar levels are high, it may be hard to convince her that high blood sugars can hurt her. Most kids live and think very much in the present, even in the moment. Those long-term complications you worry about all the time don't impress most young children very much. They're much more tuned in to today!

When you look beyond how the child feels to how she functions, how she gets along, other advantages of good blood sugar control become apparent. When your child's blood sugars are low, it's hard for her to do what she needs to do. Low blood sugars deprive the brain of the fuel required for thought. When the brain runs out of glucose—the only fuel it can use—it can't work well. It's similar to how a car starts to sputter and stall as it runs out of gas. It becomes hard to concentrate, hard to coordinate, and hard to relate to other people. If your child's blood sugar gets really low, it can even be hard to stay conscious.

Recent studies show that high blood sugars can also affect the ability to get things done. People perform tasks more slowly when they are hyperglycemic, and they make more mistakes.

Whatever the immediate advantages of good blood sugar control, you are probably even more concerned with the long-term benefits. And these benefits are undeniable. Good blood sugar control is a must for normal growth and development in children. The body needs to have plenty of energy and enough insulin in order to grow. Keeping blood sugars in control makes it possible for your child to grow and develop according to his or her own genetic blueprint.

In addition, we now know that good control is essential for minimizing the risk of long-term complications. In 1993, the results of the 10-year Diabetes Control and Complications Trial (DCCT) were released. This study was designed to answer two vital questions. First, if people treated their diabetes intensively, would their blood sugar control improve? Second, if their blood sugar did improve, would their risk of developing diabetes-related complications go down as well?

To answer these questions, people with type I diabetes were recruited from all over the country. All of them were between 13 and 39 years of age. Half of them were assigned to the intensive treatment group. They took at least three shots a day or used an insulin pump, and they tested their blood sugar at least four times a day. They also spoke and met as often as they needed to with diabetes educators—primarily nurses and dietitians. The educators provided whatever training, advice, and support people needed to become active managers of their own daily care. As a result of this emphasis on self-management, most people in the intensive treatment group learned to adjust their own insulin doses to get the best possible control between their medical visits. Their goal was to get their blood sugar as close to normal as possible without causing too much low blood sugar.

The other half of the DCCT participants received conventional treatment. They took one or two insulin shots a day, did some blood sugar testing, and had office visits every 3 months. Their goal was to control their diabetes well enough to be free of symptoms and to grow properly.

Control was monitored in both groups, using the HbA_{1c} test. The outcome was announced in June of 1993 at the American Diabetes Association Annual Meeting.

We can still remember sitting in a throng of 5,000 diabetes researchers and health-care providers when the final results were described. It was a thrilling moment. First, we learned that people in the intensive treatment group did achieve better blood sugar control. The upper limit of normal on the HbA_{1c} test used in the study was 6.05%. In the first 6 months of the study, the average HbA_{1c} of the intensive treatment group dropped from 9.0% (representing an average blood sugar of about 230 mg/dl) to 7.2% (an average blood sugar of about 155 mg/dl). It stayed at that lower level throughout the 10 years of the study. Blood sugar stayed about where it started (HbA_{1c} 9.0% and average blood sugar about 230 mg/dl) in the conventional treatment group. Adolescents in the study had slightly higher HbA_{1c} levels than adult participants in both groups; however, their results showed comparable improvements. This conclusively answered the first study question (if people treated their diabetes intensively, would their blood sugar control improve?). But did this improved control lead to fewer long-term problems?

The answer to that question was a resounding Yes! To tell the truth, most of us who gathered to hear the findings were not surprised that better blood sugar control meant fewer complications. Smaller studies and our own experience had convinced most of us of that long before this strong proof became available. What did surprise many of us, however, was how big a difference intensive treatment made. In the DCCT, intensive treatment reduced retinopathy (eye disease) by as much as 76%. Intensive treatment also reduced nephropathy (kidney disease), decreasing the development of early kidney problems (microalbuminuria) by 35% and more advanced problems (macroalbuminuria) by 56%. Neuropathy (nerve damage) was reduced by 60%.

Now we know for sure that improved blood sugar control is both possible and powerful. The DCCT has proven that complications are largely preventable through good blood sugar control in relatively young adults with type I diabetes—the type of people who were in the DCCT. Knowing that still doesn't answer the question of whether intensive treatment is the right approach for every person with diabetes. There is still some room for debate regarding groups that didn't participate in the DCCT, such as young children. Notably, no children younger than 13 participated in the study, and there were only 190 teenagers. The DCCT doesn't tell us directly what we should be doing about control in young kids. Even so, we can figure it out, using a little common sense and what we know about development and family relationships.

Should tight blood sugar control be a priority for your child? We think that the answer is yes, with certain critical qualifications.

WHAT'S REALISTIC WHEN IT COMES TO BLOOD SUGAR CONTROL IN CHILDREN?

What are the qualifications? First, you have to be realistic. Here again, the DCCT provides invaluable information. The goal for the intensive treatment group was normal blood sugar control, and every possible effort was made to achieve this goal. But even with all that effort, only 20% of the intensive treatment group ever had a normal glycohemoglobin reading during the entire study, and only 5% had normal values throughout the study. Clearly, the vast majority of people who have diabetes just can't achieve totally normal blood sugars. As the parent of a child with diabetes, this probably comes as no real surprise to you. In addition, among the teenagers in the DCCT intensive treatment group, the proportion who achieved normal glycohemoglobin readings was even lower than among the adults in the study. All this suggests that perfection, in the form of completely normal blood sugar values, is not a realistic goal when you have diabetes. And it's especially unrealistic when the person with diabetes is a child.

Years ago, a man named Lawrence Pray, who was diagnosed with diabetes in the 1940s at the age of 7, wrote a book titled *Journey of a Diabetic*. In his book, Pray offered some wise counsel: "Don't try for perfection. Try for good control, to be sure, but perfection lasts a moment, and diabetes lasts a lifetime." Perfection is impossible. If you try to achieve it, you can't succeed. Trying to achieve the impossible will only make you (and your child) frustrated and miserable. These truths apply to every person with diabetes but have special significance for children with diabetes, because their blood sugar levels often fluctuate even more dramatically than the levels of adults. And among all children, teenagers often have the hardest time with blood sugar control. We used to think this was because teenagers "act out" (the psychologist's word for misbehaving!) more than younger children or adults. Now we know that this is only part of the story. All those raging hormones of adolescence also play their part in teenage blood sugar instability. Growth hormone and stress hormones, which flow in abundance during adolescence, counteract the effects of insulin, pushing blood sugar levels up. This makes control harder to achieve during the teenage years than it was earlier in childhood, or than it will be when the teen years are past.

It's important to set realistic, as well as ambitious, goals for your child's blood sugar control. Go for control that is "good enough" rather than perfect. What is good enough? Once again, the DCCT provides the answer. Remember that the people in the DCCT who did so well still had a glycosylated hemoglobin of about 7%. That was a full percentage point above the normal range and equals an average blood sugar of about 155. Not perfect, but good enough. This "good enough" control will allow your child to feel well, grow and develop normally, and have less risk for complications. The trick is to balance the effort required to get these benefits against the family's and the child's current quality of life and against the risks that more intensive treatment brings with it.

The DCCT offers yet another boost for good (as opposed to perfect) control. Although the headlines following the release of the study's findings all trumpeted the benefits of tight control, many of us saw an even more important result. The relationship between blood sugar level and risk of complications among study participants was pretty much a straight line: the lower the blood sugar level, the lower the risk of complications, at every blood sugar level. This means that any improvement in blood sugar control will probably lead to a reduced risk of complications. You don't need to reach some specific blood glucose value before you see a benefit.

This finding cuts both ways. On the one hand, it is very encouraging, because it tells us that any lowering of blood sugar helps, even if you are starting at a level that is very high. On the other hand, many people hoped the DCCT would show that there was some threshold for the beneficial effects of improved blood sugar control. If, for example, we had found that everyone whose HbA_{1c} was below 8.0% had the same risk of developing complications, we could tell people they didn't have to try to go lower than 8%. There appears to be no such threshold. Any improvement in blood sugar makes a difference. And every improvement in blood sugar control makes a difference, whether it's from terrible to so-so, or from good to great.

RISKS OF BETTER GLUCOSE CONTROL

Every benefit in life has a certain cost. Like the athletes used to say, "No pain, no gain." But before you say, "Sign me up for that good control stuff," it's important to know the downside. You need to balance three main concerns against the benefits of good blood sugar control before making your decision. Those concerns are

- A greater risk for low blood sugars
- The chance of unwanted weight gain
- The risk of making the family crazy in trying to get perfect control

You can minimize all of these risks if you understand them.

More Low Blood Sugars

First, in the DCCT, people in the intensive treatment group had three times as much hypoglycemia as those in the standard treatment group. That should come as no surprise: when your goal is normal blood sugars, you don't have much margin for error. Think of a child walking around a deep lake. She is far more likely to fall in if she walks near the water than if she takes a path farther from the shore. In the same way, if the blood sugar is 140 and drops 80 points to 60, the child is dangerously close to a low reaction. If the blood sugar drops the same 80 points from a reading of 240, the result is a blood sugar of 160, nowhere near the low range. The closer to normal we keep the blood sugar, the more stable and exact control must be to prevent low blood sugars. In a sense, there is less room for error: less room for the sometimes surprising shifts in blood sugar that happen because of factors we don't understand or can't control. Because of this risk, the researchers involved in the DCCT specifically stated that intensive therapy with the goal of normal blood sugars may not be right for children under the age of 13, and especially under the age of 7 (because of the greater risk to brain development posed by hypoglycemia in the very young child).

Hypoglycemia (which we discuss more fully in Chapter 7) is a special problem for children. For one thing, young children may have trouble recognizing when they are low and communicating what's going on. In addition, severe hypoglycemia, especially if it is frequent, can affect the developing brains of very young children (those under the age of 7 or so). When a person is hypoglycemic, her brain is starved for fuel. In very young children, the fuel is needed not just for immediate functioning but for brain development as well. Before you run off in a panic, keep in mind that the effects are probably restricted to young children, and that the magnitude of impact is hard to measure with any accuracy. Still, this concern reinforces the importance of not pushing for the lowest possible blood sugar levels.

Unwanted Weight Gain

The second potential drawback of tight control—weight gain—also was documented in the DCCT. Those in the intensive treatment group gained an average of 10 pounds more over the course of the study than those in the conventional treatment group. There are several possible reasons for this. One of them has to do with the blood sugar level itself. When blood sugar is high (above about 180 for most people), sugar ends up in the urine. The sugar in the urine contains calories that the body never had a chance to use. That's why weight loss is often a sign that diabetes control needs improvement. When control does improve, the body hangs on to all the calories eaten, just as it does in people who don't have diabetes. If control is good and you eat more food than you need, you gain weight. (In Chapter 9, we talk about the way some young people—mostly young women—use this fact to control their weight).

Another cause for weight gain on intensive therapy has to do with those extra episodes of low blood sugar. If there are extra lows, each one has to be treated with food, leading to extra calorie intake. This is another good reason for making the prevention of low blood sugars a high priority.

Also, in an effort to get blood sugar in excellent control, the doctor or the family may sometimes overadjust the insulin. If people take more insulin than they really need, they then have to eat to "feed" that insulin to avoid lows. It's another way in which people can end up eating more food than they really need. As long as control is good, those extra calories will get socked away as body fat.

Finally, when people get very skilled at the intensive style of treatment that produces great blood sugar control, they generally follow more liberal meal plans than people on more traditional treatment regimens. They learn how to eat sweets and other favorite foods just like the rest of us, while still keeping the blood sugar in control. Eating more favorite high-calorie foods equals more likelihood to gain weight. Keep in mind that gaining some weight is normal when blood sugar control improves from a poor level. It happens because good control allows the body to correct dehydration and replace muscle and fat that were burned for energy while control was poor. However, if undesired weight gain continues, the diabetes team should check out the entire management plan, including insulin doses, food intake, and the occurrence of low blood sugars.

Letting Diabetes Control the Family

The third and final risk of going after great blood sugar control is the danger of forgetting other goals important to the family and its members, the danger of letting diabetes control the family. As we've said, the most basic way to combat this possibility is to remember that perfect blood sugar control is simply not possible. In Chapters 13 and 14, we describe important tactics for keeping the family and its members sane.

Given all of this information, you and your child need to work out the diabetes treatment regimen and goals for control that make sense for your family. Before we go on to offer some guidelines for making these decisions, we want to mention one more fact to consider. Much of our motivation in working for good blood sugar control is avoiding complications. Most complications appear after many years of diabetes. That's what frightens many of us who have children with diabetes: they have so many years to live with their disease. But there is some evidence that during the years before adolescence, the "complications clock" ticks more slowly than it does in later years. Some researchers estimate that every adult year with diabetes contributes doubly to the development of complications, compared with a year of childhood with the disease. This may help you feel a little less pressured as you work out an effective plan for helping your child manage her diabetes.

We can't tell you exactly what your own goals and plan will be. Each family must answer that question for itself. Your best plan depends on your personalities, lifestyle, values, and resources. When you find your answer, diabetes will assume its proper priority in your family's life: important but not all-consuming. Finding that balance is a repeated process for most families. They get there for a while and then something changes that puts the diabetes back in the driver's seat again. When that happens, finding the balance again is very important to everyone. It makes life more enjoyable in the short run, to be sure, but finding the balance is also very important to your child's long-term success in dealing with diabetes.

BALANCING BLOOD SUGAR CONTROL WITH OTHER IMPORTANT GOALS

Here's the goal: raising a normal (as much like other kids as possible), healthy, emotionally strong, independent child who will be able to deal with all the challenges life presents—those that come from diabetes and those that don't. As you know only too well, working toward that goal is a difficult balancing act. You can't tilt too far one way or the other. If you put all of your energy into trying to control your child's blood sugars, other essential aspects of life will be sacrificed. If you let your child live as if she didn't have diabetes, her health will be at risk.

The situation is complicated by the fact that you may feel your child is so concerned with being normal that all the responsibility for seeing to it that she follows her diabetes regimen is left to you. As a result, it may seem you are constantly arguing, angry, frustrated, and disappointed. There has to be a better way, and fortunately, there is. To find that way, you have to start by understanding that good blood sugar control actually goes hand-in-hand with emotional health and independence. All appearances to the contrary, it's actually a package deal: you either get both or you get neither. To get both, you and your child must work together. You must cooperate, recognizing and respecting some important facts.

Find Unique Solutions and Goals for Your Family

First among these is a fact we mentioned earlier: your family is unique. Any workable plan for living with diabetes has to take into account your family's schedules, strengths, and vulnerabilities; the personalities of its members; and the support you have from family and friends for coping with day-to-day stresses. The best plan will be one thing if you are a single, working parent with several children to care for and no family or friends available to lighten your load. It will be quite another if you are a two-parent family with only one child and lots of outside support.

Help Your Child Learn to Care for Herself

Another fact important to balancing sanity with diabetes control involves your role in your child's care. You might think you are responsible for controlling your child's blood sugar, but you are not. Your real responsibility, if you want your child to have a healthy, happy life, is to help her learn to control her own blood sugar. When you take responsibility for solving all the problems involved in managing your child's diabetes, two bad things happen. First, you deprive her of the critically important opportunity of learning how to solve her own problems. She will need that skill throughout her life, and it can only be developed through practice. Second, when you take full responsibility for controlling your child's diabetes, she is left with only one way to exert her own control—by resisting you. The result is almost always a deadlock, with everyone miserable. The following story illustrates a more effective approach.

Sally was 7 years old when she was diagnosed with diabetes, just a few weeks before the winter holiday season. Among the many painful adjustments the family faced was the prospect of giving up the precious tradition of baking Christmas cookies. Sally's mom was convinced that baking the cookies would be courting disaster, because Sally would insist on gorging herself on them, as she had in the past. Sally's mom was taking responsibility for controlling her daughter's blood sugars. And who could blame her? But the result of her efforts was very sad: Sally felt deprived and resentful. Her mother felt both guilty for denying her daughter and angry at the same time. The rest of the family just didn't know what to do.

When Sally and her mom brought up this dilemma on a visit to the pediatric diabetes clinic where Sally received her treatment, the counselor suggested an experiment. Instead of Mom taking responsibility for solving the problem, Sally should be given the responsibility. This seemed like a pretty radical idea to both of them, but they were willing to give it a try. The counselor described the rules of the experiment. Sally could suggest any solution to the problem that appealed to her. Mom then could accept the suggestion, offer a countersuggestion, or say no. She had to promise not to put Sally down for her suggestions, no matter how outrageous they might seem to her. She had to say no matter-of-factly, in a way that encouraged Sally to come up with another suggestion. If Mom heard a suggestion that she felt had the kernel of a good idea, but not the whole answer, she could suggest a modification to Sally. Then Sally could either say yes, no, or offer her own counterproposal.

Sally and her mom quickly got the hang of the experiment, the essence of which is working cooperatively to solve a family problem. After offering a few possible solutions that her mom turned down, Sally suggested that she be allowed to have one cookie a day during the holidays. Her mother was reluctant to accept this idea because she feared a continuing battle over the issue. She just couldn't believe Sally would accept her daily cookie and not whine and moan for more. Sally, for her part, was certain that she could accept the limit, adding that one cookie a day was better than none.

The counselor saw the possibility of a workable solution on the table and jumped in to ask Sally what she would suggest as a consequence if she found herself unable to live with her agreement. Sally immediately answered, "We could take all the rest of the cookies and give them to the neighbors." At this, her mom laughed and said she was willing to give it a try. To check out one last potential flaw in the plan, the counselor asked Sally's mother what the rest of the family would say if their beloved cookies suddenly disappeared halfway through the holidays. She laughed again and said, "I'll just make it clear to them from the start what the deal is. Either we'll all have cookies, or none of us will."

This approach works because you assume your proper responsibility and allow your child to do the same. It's your child's responsibility to learn how to control her diabetes. And it's your responsibility to help her learn and to protect her from hurting herself in the process. In our experience, this approach works, even with children as young as 4 or 5.

Let's say your 5-year-old daughter was looking forward to ice cream for dessert. You test her blood before dinner and she's 320. Your natural response is, "No ice cream tonight!" Then what happens? Your child gets upset in whatever way she does—whining, pouting, yelling—and you get upset, too. All too often the real issue, how to manage your child's food when her blood sugar level is high, gets lost in the ensuing uproar.

Even a 5-year-old child can begin to solve the real problem. You can tell her what the problem is: it's not safe to let her blood sugars go any higher, and the ice cream might do that. Then you can ask her what she thinks the right approach might be. Remember the way Sally and her mother worked together. If your child suggests eating the ice cream anyway, you can tell her that won't work, and encourage her to think of another idea. If she gets frustrated and says she can't think of anything or if she gets upset and says she just won't have any, you can tell her you're sorry she can't think of anything that would work. If you have any ideas yourself, you could offer them.

When this approach is used consistently, kids quickly get the idea that they can have something they want if they can solve the problem safely. Your child might suggest extra insulin to correct the high blood sugar and cover the ice cream, keeping the blood sugar from going higher. Or she might suggest some exercise after dinner and before dessert. Or she might suggest saving the ice cream for tomorrow. Whatever she suggests, you can accept, offer a counterproposal, or say no. If she offers a solution that appeals to you, a few extra units of Regular insulin, for instance, you can even take the problem-solving lesson to the next level and ask her how many units she thinks she needs. If she says three units but you think two would be better, you can suggest she start with two and that when you test her blood at bedtime, you both can tell how good your guess was. That will give you both information for the next time you face the same problem. Even more importantly, it will give your child the experience she will need when she begins to face these decisions on her own.

And the time when she will have to do so is just around the corner. Even if your child is only 5 or 6 years old, you will only be able to control her blood sugars for a few more years. After that, for better or for worse, she will begin making her own decisions. By the time she is 14 or 15, she will be managing most aspects of her diabetes herself. Start now with a new, more effective approach to managing your child's diabetes. Don't try to control your child's blood sugars. Help her learn how to control her own.

DEAL WITH YOUR FEARS ABOUT TRYING THIS APPROACH

To take the approach we recommend, you need to deal with your own fears. "Aren't you being an irresponsible parent?" "Won't your child's control go haywire?" Our answers to these questions are no and no. You are being a highly responsible parent when you prepare her to solve the daily problems she will face throughout her life with diabetes. You are teaching her the most valuable lesson of all: she can do anything she wants to do, as long as she can figure out how to do it safely. Your child's control will not worsen if she learns to take responsibility for her own care. While she is young, you are still there to say yes or no to any particular proposal she might offer, so she is protected in that way. And as she gets older and is making more of her decisions independently, she will be prepared to make those decisions wisely. She won't be left with those all-or-nothing choices of either feeling deprived or letting her blood sugars go where they will. All too often, young people don't learn how to solve diabetes-related problems when they are young because their parents insist on trying—however unsuccessfully—to solve all the problems for them.

CONTINUE TO WORK WITH YOUR OLDER CHILD

Our fundamental point here is that it can't be and shouldn't be only your responsibility to control your child's blood sugars. On the other hand, all the responsibility for diabetes management shouldn't fall to your child either. Neither extreme works. Just as even the youngest child can begin to take part in diabetes-related problem-solving, even the 18-year-old needs some help and support at times. The old approach to diabetes care for children was for parents to control their children until the kids reached a certain age, usually about 10 years old, and then turn over all responsibility to the child. We've talked about the need for cooperation in the early years. Now let's talk about the importance of maintaining this approach as your child gets older.

Until about 10 years ago, independence in diabetes care was seen as a sign of maturity, a sign the child was beginning to take responsibility for her own diabetes. Parents and health-care providers often discussed early independence as if it were an achievement, a sign of responsibility, maturity, and intelligence, like early reading. But recent research shows something quite different. These studies show that diabetes is not just a child's disease. It's a family disease. Diabetes affects the lives of everyone in the family. It affects family activities, routines, demands, worries, and emergencies. Research points to two things that the families of children whose diabetes is in control have in common. First, the children in these families—regardless of their age—have continuing support with diabetes management tasks from their parents. Second, there is less conflict in these families than there is in families where kids are in poorer control.

We recommend that you don't focus on your child's age alone when you think about what she should be doing when it comes to caring for her diabetes. Even though age used to be the standard, we now know that age guidelines don't work. One reason they don't is that there is almost always a big difference between a child's physical capacity to master a task and the cognitive and emotional maturity required to carry out the task on a continuing basis. Not recognizing this difference is the source of tremendous frustration for the parents of a child with diabetes: you know she can do her blood sugar tests, so why doesn't she?

Gary Ingersoll and his colleagues at the University of Indiana conducted a study that tells us a lot about the pitfalls of assuming that kids with diabetes will assume responsibility for their own care just because they are old enough to physically master the required tasks. Ingersoll found that many of the parents he studied withdrew from the process of helping their children adjust insulin doses. But the kids didn't assume the responsibility themselves. Instead, the whole insulin adjustment process simply slipped between the cracks.

Another problem with turning over responsibility for diabetes management based solely on your child's age is the fact that not all kids the same age have the same capacities. Temperament and other individual differences powerfully affect the way children adapt to diabetes or to any other major life challenge. If you don't take your child's individuality into account and continue to provide the diabetes management support she needs, you will both end up with unnecessary feelings of frustration and failure.

Yet another problem with age guidelines for independent self-care is the fact that guidelines don't take into account external stresses or special needs. Family problems, learning disabilities, and a wide range of other factors must be considered when developing a workable diabetes care plan for your family.

There are some teenagers who seem to adamantly resist taking responsibility for their own diabetes care. If your child acts this way, you need to stay as involved as possible and move slowly as you help her move toward independence. If things get especially rocky, talk to your child's health-care team about the possibility of family counseling, preferably with a professional experienced in working with teens who have diabetes.

BALANCING THE BENEFITS OF CONTROL WITH THE FAMILY'S OTHER NEEDS

As we pointed out before, we believe that the most important task facing all parents is to raise emotionally healthy and independent children. That task may be even more important when the child in question has diabetes. After all, we know that the child with diabetes will face special challenges all through life. We know that she will need strength, discipline, self-confidence, and great diabetes management skills to deal with the challenges presented by diabetes over the years. If a child grows up observing and participating actively in a balanced and cooperative approach to dealing with diabetes, she is more likely to carry the same attitudes and behaviors into adult life. Making diabetes the center of family fights by overdoing parental control or giving up in despair shows the child ways of handling her diabetes that will continue to cause her problems throughout her life. Raising a child with diabetes who is healthy in every way is not easy, but it is possible. You need to set personal "good enough" blood sugar goals appropriate to your child's age and ability and to your family's values, supports, and resources. Then you need to help your child learn to take care of herself well enough to achieve them.

You can't totally ignore the gorilla at the symphony (see **Introduction: What Diabetes Can Do To Families**), but by sharing responsibility for management in age-appropriate ways, you can keep that gorilla in his place so you can enjoy the process of raising your kids.

THE BOTTOM LINE

1. Blood sugar control is very important, in both the short and the long term.
2. Blood sugar goals should be both ambitious and realistic. Goals will change throughout your child's growing-up years.
3. Your responsibility is helping your child learn to control her own blood sugars.
4. The child who learns how to control her own blood sugars will be more independent and emotionally healthy and will achieve better glucose control.
5. A problem-solving approach, based on asking good questions, will help your child learn how to control her blood sugars.
6. You will have both hits and misses in diabetes management. Learn from both.
7. Begin working on diabetes management with your child at an early age and continue through the teen years.

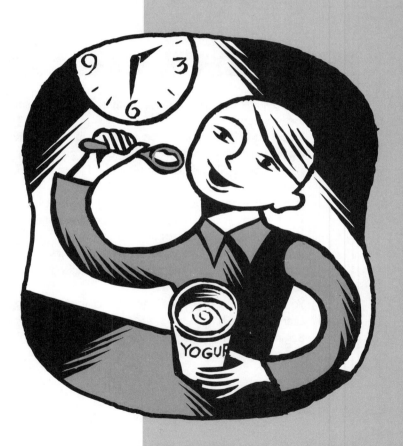

"You're telling me Jared needs to eat six times a day?"

Why Kids Need Snacks and What to Prepare

Diabetes aside, small frequent feedings work well for most children.

Jared's mother and father impressed us from the start with their can-do attitude about diabetes. Busy people with lots of commitments, they approach diabetes with the same discipline and organization that they apply to work, sports, and family activities. The day they got the news about Jared's diabetes, they asked a lot of questions. They took careful notes as first one member of the diabetes team and then another laid out the basics of diabetes care. Amazingly, only one thing about the treatment approach seemed to bother them at that first session: our recommendation that 7-year-old Jared eat three daily snacks between meals and at bedtime.

"I don't believe in eating between meals," Jared's father explained. "My aunts are always noshing on something, and they're way too heavy for their own good. We eat good, substantial meals, and it's always been enough to carry us through. Jared's doing fine, and he hasn't eaten between meals since he started school."

111

A 7-year-old child who didn't eat between meals sounded like a pretty unique creature to us. Diabetes aside, small frequent feedings work well for most children. Little stomachs coupled with high energy demands mean that most children are ready to eat at least every 3 or 4 hours while they're awake. They need more frequent stoking of their energy furnaces than the usual schedule of adult meals can provide. Most kids can't last from lunch at noon till dinner at 6 P.M. without eating again. And the 13-hour gap between a 6 P.M. dinner and a 7 A.M. breakfast is more than just about any small stomach can bear. It's not a matter of discipline, as Jared's dad seemed to think. It's a matter of physiology.

We began by explaining that snacks are normal for all kids. We also could assure the family that snacks composed of the same good foods they were eating for meals would be a positive nutritional change, not a negative one. The excess weight that Jared's folks were worried about wouldn't be a problem, because we weren't talking about *adding* three substantial snacks to what Jared was already eating. We were recommending dividing the same amount of food up into a larger number of feedings. The same amount of food would do a better job of controlling Jared's appetite and his blood sugar if it were spread out more evenly through the day.

This is a very different situation than the one that Dad seemed to fear. It's true that couch-potato kids (and elderly aunts!) who lay around gorging on bags of chips and snack cakes are at high risk for becoming overly heavy. Their lack of activity is as much to blame for this as their food choices. (It should not come as a surprise that skinny people eat junk too. It's just that observers don't get upset about it, as they seem to when they see a heavy person eating chips and cookies.)

Mom, being a bit closer to Jared's actual eating behavior than Dad on most days, finally set the record straight. "Well, honey, you know he almost always does have a sandwich and milk when he comes home from school," she offered. "And what about the popcorn or yogurt we all have while we're watching TV at night? I'd say that's a snack too."

Her remarks made it clear that they were already well over halfway toward the meal and snack pattern that was going to be most helpful for Jared. And it was a relief to learn that he was really a normal kid after all: he was already eating five times a day. The changes we were suggesting weren't going to be as drastic as the family first feared. And, best of all, he hadn't been running around hungry for years because of his aunts' indiscretions!

THE SPECIAL ROLE OF SNACKS IN DIABETES

While snacks are normal for all kids, they take on special significance in diabetes. Most people are aware of their importance in preventing low blood sugars between meals and during exercise. But did you know that they also help prevent high blood sugars by distributing food more evenly throughout the day, making a better match with the action of our current forms of injected insulin? And how about this: snacks can be your secret weapon for avoiding rigid meal plans while still keeping blood sugar under control!

WHY SNACKS ARE NEEDED TO PREVENT LOW BLOOD SUGAR

The need for snacks to prevent low blood sugar between meals, overnight, and during exercise is caused by differences between the body's own insulin and injected insulin. The bodies of people who don't have diabetes always produce exactly the right amount of insulin automatically, anytime they decide to eat. They also get small steady amounts between meals and overnight to keep the blood sugar level perfectly balanced. And they automatically get even less during exercise to help the body release its own sugar supply to provide extra fuel. A great system!

Figure 6.1 shows how much the action of injected insulin differs from that normal picture. Notice the dotted line representing injected insulin. The lines represent an insulin pattern that's used very commonly for kids: two injections a day of a combination of Regular and NPH or Lente insulin. The places where it is much higher than the solid line representing the body's own insulin reflect the times when risk for low blood sugar is greatest. Notice that the peak (greatest action) of the body's insulin is very sharp and occurs very quickly after eating. The peaks of the injected insulins, on the other hand, are much more blunt, last longer, and occur later.

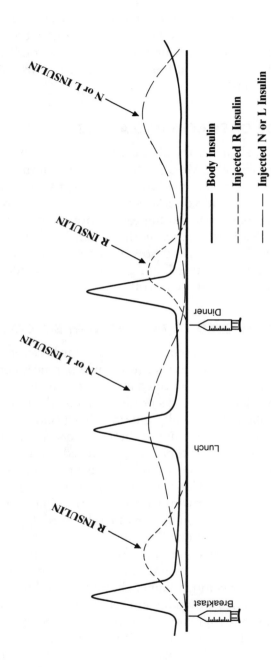

FIGURE 6.1

Too much injected insulin is still hanging around when the body would normally have very small amounts—principally before and between meals and overnight. If food isn't eaten at those times, the result will be a falling blood sugar level. That's why skipping or delaying meals or snacks is the most common cause of low blood sugar. The same thing can happen during exercise, because we're not able to take away insulin that was injected earlier in the day. (See Chapter 8 for more information about managing exercise.)

HOW SNACKS HELP PREVENT HIGH BLOOD SUGAR

Having high blood sugar after eating is a problem for just about everybody with diabetes. Those same blunted peaks of Regular, NPH, and Lente insulin that increase risk for between-meal low blood sugar also contribute to those high blood sugars right after meals. The problem occurs because these insulins don't begin to act very soon after they're injected. Unless there's quite a delay—as much as 45 minutes, depending on the dose and the injection site—between the shot and the meal, blood sugar from the meal beats the rising level of insulin to the punch. Trying to get a long enough delay between the insulin injection and eating can help a lot, but it's a very hard thing for most people to do.

The fact is, most people take their insulin 30 minutes or less before they eat. Sluggish insulin taken that close to the meal just can't handle a whole lot of food at once. That's where snacks come in. By making meals a bit lighter and moving the difference into between-meal and bedtime snacks, insulin demand is more closely matched to the actual availability of the insulin. This results in fewer highs and fewer lows, producing more stable blood sugar control, thanks to regular snacks.

SNACKS CAN RELEASE YOU FROM THE GRIP OF RIGID MEAL PLANS

The Cartwright family was struggling with their son Joe's variable appetite. He was usually eager to eat everything on the carefully laid out exchange meal and snack plan. It's just that he didn't often want it when the plan said he should be eating it. A lot of encouragement and vigilance went into trying to get Joe to eat the three Starch Exchanges at breakfast every day, but eat only one at the morning snack; to not eat fruit with lunch, but always take one Fruit Exchange with the afternoon snack; to always drink 12 oz. of milk at dinner, but stop at half a cup with the bedtime snack.

The whole family was working awfully hard to stick to the plan, but by their estimate, they were only getting about 50% of it done as printed on the meal plan. They were tired of fighting over every meal and snack, and who could blame them? Here's what we recommended to them.

THINK OF THE MEAL PLAN IN TIME BLOCKS

You can greatly reduce the "rigid meal plan blues" by thinking of the meal plan in time blocks instead of as separate meals and snacks. One meal and one snack are covered by each of the insulins acting during the day. Because of the rather broad peaks of these insulins, it's possible to think of all the food covered by a given insulin dose as one block. If we do this, food can be moved back and forth between the meal and snack within a given time block without jeopardizing insulin coverage or blood sugar control.

To help you see exactly how this works, look at the two-injection mixed-insulin plan illustrated in Figure 6.1. On this insulin schedule, the morning Regular insulin lasts from breakfast until just before lunch. The morning NPH or Lente covers from lunch until just before dinner. The evening Regular insulin covers from dinner until bedtime, and the evening NPH or Lente covers from bedtime until just before breakfast. If your child takes three injections, he takes his NPH or Lente insulin at bedtime instead of dinnertime. It still covers from bedtime until breakfast, but the peak action takes place closer to dawn than what is shown in the illustration.

Table 6.1 shows how little Joe Cartwright's unpredictable appetite can be dealt with by using the time block method. The first column shows Joe's usual pattern of food intake based on his diabetes meal plan, expressed in grams of carbohydrate. The second column shows how it might divide out differently on a

TABLE 6.1 Using Time Blocks to Adjust for Changes in Hunger

	Meal Plan	Day 1: Not Hungry	Day 2: Extra Hungry
	57 g carbohydrate	**36 g carbohydrate**	**72 g carbohydrate**
Breakfast	cereal with 4 oz. milk 1/2 banana 1 slice toast 4 oz. milk to drink	cereal with 4 oz. milk 1/2 banana	2 slices toast with peanut butter 1 whole banana 8 oz. milk
	30 g carbohydrate	**51 g carbohydrate**	**15 g carbohydrate**
Morning Snack	8 oz. carton milk 1 cup strawberries	2/3 cup grape juice peanut butter crackers	small can juice celery and peanuts

day when his appetite is not so hearty at breakfast. On that kind of day, Mom can save some of the carbohydrate grams usually eaten at breakfast and add them to the morning snack. This almost amounts to reversing the order of the snack and the breakfast. Joe's mother didn't think he'd be hungry for a full meal at snack time either, so she offered more concentrated sources of carbohydrate. This way he gets everything he needs in a smaller package: 2/3 cup of grape juice (30 grams of carbohydrate) instead of a cup of strawberries (15 grams of carbohydrate). He gets the same insulin coverage with fewer calories and less bulk.

The third column shows how Joe's carbohydrate allowance would be divided up on a day when he was feeling extra hungry when he got up. Carbohydrate-containing foods were borrowed from the snack in order to satisfy his morning appetite. Food can be moved around within the breakfast-to-lunchtime block in many different combinations. But regardless of exactly when he eats it during the block, he's still eating the same total amount of food relative to the same total amount of insulin. In column three, the snack is smaller than usual, because he ate part of it at breakfast time. The snack has been filled out with things that don't raise blood sugar, such as raw vegetables and peanuts.

The time block strategy can also be used when Junior gets himself ousted from the dinner table for acting like a little Philistine. Remember those parent-child job descriptions? The child gets to decide how much he's going to eat of the available food, but he has to follow the family's rules for mealtime behavior. Maybe you had to ask him to leave the table when he made that really rude noise for the third time. If his blood sugar was on the low side before dinner, you might be generous and let him take his milk with him when he leaves the table.

Rely on the time block system to keep things under control, allowing you to parent the child. When it comes time for the bedtime snack, add the equivalent of what was missed at dinner to the regular snack. Offer it in a more concentrated form, if you think that's necessary. But the child may be hungry enough by then to just eat the dinner leftovers. It's probably smartest to offer foods that you can always rely on your child eating. If it's reasonably important that the child eat a substantial bedtime snack because he had to leave the dinner table after eating very little, avoid any temptation to use the snack for a power play. Lay off things you know he doesn't like. Offer some of his preferred foods instead, reducing the chance of another hassle.

As it has for many families, using the time block method gave the Cartwright family a new perspective on how to use that little printed meal plan and made it much easier for them to follow the parent and child job descriptions.

WHAT MAKES A GOOD SNACK?

Anything that makes a good meal also makes a good snack. To get the best appetite control and most stable blood sugar levels, offer a combination of carbohydrate, protein, and small amounts of fat. Since most of the protein sources we eat—meat, milk, cheese, peanut butter, etc.—naturally contain some fat, it's seldom necessary to add fat separately.

Snacks containing only carbohydrate (like fruit, for example) immediately satisfy hunger and release blood sugar quickly, but they won't support blood sugar or control hunger for very long. Snacks composed of only protein and fat (like beef jerky) aren't immediately satisfying and don't release much glucose in the first couple of hours after they're eaten to provide insulin coverage. However, the protein and fat tend to provide good long-term appetite control (so the kids are not coming back an hour later for another snack), and they provide better protection against low blood sugar several hours after

TABLE 6.2 The Best Snacks Provide Both Carbohydrate and Protein

Carbohydrate Source	Protein Source
Crackers	String cheese
Bread	Peanut butter
Fresh apple	Reduced-fat cheddar cheese
Dry cereal	Low-fat milk
Hot-air popcorn	Sugar-free hot chocolate
Fruit	Cottage cheese
Bread (for sandwich)	Sliced chicken, meat, or cheese
Tortilla	Scrambled egg whites w/salsa

eating than pure carbohydrate does. When you combine carbohydrate and protein in meals and snacks, you get the best of both worlds for most snacking needs. You achieve appetite control that is both immediate and relatively long-lasting. And you get sustained insulin coverage that begins soon and stretches all the way until the next meal or snack.

Table 6.2 shows some of the combinations that work well. Substitute similar foods that your child prefers if these Starch, Fruit, or Protein selections aren't appealing. If you and the kids start getting bored with snacks, we suggest getting *The Joy of Snacks,* by Nancy Cooper (available from the American Diabetes Association). It has more great snack ideas than most of us would get around to in a lifetime.

SPECIAL TIPS FOR BEDTIME SNACKS

The purpose of bedtime snacks in diabetes is to protect against low blood sugar during sleep. The most common time for low blood sugar reactions is 2 to 3 A.M. This high level of risk is related to three things. First, insulin is much more effective at that time of the night because of normal variations in body hormones. Second, it's difficult to adjust NPH or Lente injected before the meal to get the insulin level low enough between 2 and 3 A.M. and still avoid high fasting blood sugar the next morning. Third, most people snack at least several hours before the time when overnight lows tend to happen. Therefore, to protect against those overnight lows, we need "time release" bedtime snacks that provide glucose several hours after eating. Some snacks do that and others don't.

To put a floor under falling overnight blood sugar, a snack must contain foods that release their glucose to the bloodstream slowly. As we've said, protein and fat accomplish this quite well. Some people think this is because protein and fat are digested fairly slowly, so any glucose they produce enters the bloodstream several hours after eating. Other people think it's because having protein or fat in a meal or snack slows down the body's digestion of the carbohydrate it contains. Either way, having substantial protein and/or fat in a meal or snack seems to support blood sugar for a much longer time than if carbohydrate is eaten alone. Protein and fat are provided by meat, fish, poultry, cheese, milk, yogurt, and beans. "Lente carbohydrate" refers to those carbohydrate-containing foods that seem to release their sugar over a longer period of time. We've had the best results with foods such as oatmeal, barley, pasta, pizza, beans, and cornstarch.

Cornstarch can be stirred into other items, such as yogurt, sugar-free pudding, or peanut butter. Start with a teaspoon of cornstarch (5 grams of carbohydrate) and increase a teaspoon at a time up to a tablespoon until blood sugars stay in a desirable range overnight. You'll need to use those lovely 2 to 3 A.M. blood tests to see how your experiments with different bedtime snacks are working. Table 6.3 has some examples of specific snacks that have worked well for children who were having problems with low blood sugar in the middle of the night.

A very common alternative to putting so much effort into the bedtime snack is to move the dinnertime NPH or Lente insulin to bedtime or to change the predinner insulin to Ultralente. This moves the peak of the insulin away from the critical 2 to 3 A.M. time frame and closer to dawn, where it can do a better job of controlling fasting blood sugar. Of course, the first solution means another injection, but if that's acceptable, it can work very well. This is even possible for very young children with early bedtimes. The NPH or Lente is given at the parents' bedtime. Many children won't even wake up when this is done.

And don't forget to have your child brush his teeth after the bedtime snack. Diabetes is associated with a much higher

TABLE 6.3 Bedtime Snacks Likely to Prevent Overnight Lows

- Pizza and diet soda
- Oatmeal and raisins with milk
- Bean, split pea, lentil, or barley soup
- Bean burrito with cheese
- Sugar-free pudding or yogurt with cornstarch added

risk for gum disease and cavities, so good dental hygiene is especially important.

TIMING OF SNACKS

When you control the timing as well as the type of food available for snacks, you can greatly increase the chances that snacks will satisfy the child's hunger and help with blood sugar control. Midway between meals is best for most youngsters. If snacks are available too soon after a meal, the child may refuse them because he's not hungry yet. Or it may encourage him to skip or "cherry pick" at the meal, holding out for more preferred foods at the snack. Having the snack halfway between the meals makes it more likely that he'll be hungry for the snack—but not too hungry. Holding off snack time until a child is famished raises the likelihood of fussiness and arguments.

Spreading meals and snacks out pretty evenly through the day also provides good insulin coverage, reducing the likelihood of extreme highs and lows in the blood sugar. Two snacks are okay if it's a really long stretch between meals. If this happens, make the last snack all or mostly all carbohydrate—fruit, juice, or crackers, for example. These foods are not as likely to stick around long enough to interfere with the child's appetite for the coming meal. They also have a somewhat shorter effect on the blood sugar, which is desirable, because you're probably going to be checking the blood sugar before the next meal.

We understand that sometimes snacks cannot be eaten at the planned times. Maybe the drive home from school took an extra 45 minutes because of a traffic jam. Or maybe the teacher kept the whole class after school. Perhaps your child forgot to take his snack with him when he went out bike riding and returned home famished less than an hour before dinner. These and other things happen. It's called life. What you do about delayed snacks, of course, depends on the situation. What's the blood sugar? How long is it until the next meal? Is the child hungry?

Here are some options. If the delayed snack produced low blood sugar, treat the low blood sugar first. Then give the planned snack. Depending on how low the glucose fell, you may need to give more than was planned originally for the snack. If the blood sugar is in the desired range, just go ahead and give the snack. But if the next meal is coming up fairly soon, you may want to eliminate some or all of the fat and protein from the snack to help make sure that the child will be hungry for the coming meal. If the blood glucose is high, you can reduce the amount of carbohydrate in the snack to prevent driving the blood sugar up even higher.

WHAT IF BLOOD SUGARS ARE TOO HIGH AFTER SNACKS?

Blood sugars that are consistently above your child's target range before a meal can be dealt with in several ways. The best choice depends on your preferences and the exact cause of the high readings. First, make sure that you're not testing too close to the snack. (There are, undoubtedly, differences in your goals for after-meal and before-meal blood sugars. For example, many people try to keep before-meal blood sugars between 70 and 120 or 70 and 140, but goals for after-meal blood sugars are more likely to be less than 160, 180, or even 200.) If a test is done less than 2 hours after eating, it's very likely that the glucose reading will be on the high side, but hopefully not higher than the after-meal goal. This can happen even if the total amount of food is well matched by the insulin dose. Changing the timing of the snack relative to the insulin may be the simplest way to improve the blood glucose.

If the snack was eaten at least a couple of hours before a high test, you need to decide whether the situation calls for changing the food or changing the insulin. If you feel that the total amount of food in the time block (breakfast plus the morning snack, for example) is right for your child's appetite, one option is to increase the insulin dose to better cover that amount of food. (See Chapter 4 for some general guidelines on insulin adjustments for high blood sugar and for variations in food intake.) You could also cut down on the amount of carbohydrate by either moving a starch or fruit serving into the previous meal or reducing the total amount of carbohydrate. This can be accomplished by simply eliminating a serving of a high-carbohydrate food or by substituting foods that have less effect on blood sugar. The best approach depends on your child's appetite and food preferences, as well as his overall nutritional intake.

For example, 8-year-old Linda's blood sugar had been around 200 mg/dl before lunch for 3 days in a row. She had her snack about 10 A.M. and lunch at 12:30 P.M., so the reading wasn't related to testing too soon after the snack. She was having two starch servings, one fruit, and one milk at breakfast and two more starches and a milk at her morning snack. She and her mom talked about whether she would like to make the snack smaller and eat more at breakfast or just cut down a bit. She said breakfast was just right. She didn't want to make that any bigger by moving some of her snack into breakfast. On the other hand, she didn't really want to make the snack any smaller. She didn't think one starch and a milk would be enough to carry her all the way until lunch. Linda and her mom decided to change her snack to one starch, one meat, and one milk. This would provide less carbohydrate, but about the same total amount of food. She could have a cracker and cheese snack pack or half a peanut butter sandwich with her milk. She was happy with the change because it satisfied her appetite and improved her blood sugar before lunch.

Occasionally, a child will want to eat such substantial snacks that it's actually necessary to add a small extra dose of insulin to cover it. This is most often an issue with the after-school snack. Whether it's a morning injection of NPH or a noontime injection of Regular that's being relied on to cover the afternoon snack, it's possible that there may not be enough around by 3 or 4 in the afternoon to handle a really big snack. Some kids are so active after school with play or sports that this is never an issue. Other kids are famished because of hard physical play and want to eat everything in sight when they get home. If and when your youngster has high blood sugars following really substantial snacks, a very small extra insulin bolus may be needed to keep things in check. The dose will probably be much smaller than what you would give for the same amount of food if it was eaten at a meal, because there's still some insulin hanging around from the previous injection. Caution is doubly important if there's going to be another shot in a couple of hours or so at the next meal. If the child resists adding another shot, try changing the composition of the snack. Less carbohydrate with more protein, fat, or fiber may produce better blood sugar control, eliminating the need for a booster insulin injection. Yet another option is using Ultralente insulin in the morning. Its longer activity may give better coverage for afternoon snacks than morning NPH or Lente.

One of us had a young patient named Geri who liked to have a sandwich, a bag of chips, milk, and a cookie after school. This was basically a second lunch, and because it came late in the afternoon, the tail of her morning NPH just wasn't getting the job done. We tried increasing the morning dose, but that just tended to make Geri low before she got out of school. Next we tried a two-unit booster of Regular insulin before she ate her snack. That wouldn't have been anywhere near enough insulin for that amount of food at a regular meal, but it worked great for her afternoon snack. If your child is having this type of problem, be sure to check with your health-care provider before adding any extra insulin shots to his schedule. This approach may or may not be a good idea in his particular circumstances.

HOW DO WE GET THE KIDS TO CARRY SNACKS?

When children are small, of course, most of their snacks will be eaten at home. But even toddlers will have occasional outings to the park or other places that call for carrying snacks along. And older kids will be taking most of their snacks away from home. The questions of where to stash them and how to carry them (and get the kids to carry their own) are important.

Avoid becoming that well-known (at least in diabetes circles) superhero: Simple Sugar Woman (or Man)! You know, the one who leaps over benches full of Little Leaguers at a single bound to give Johnny a box of juice when she sees him go pale from her vantage point in the bleachers.

Carrying his own snacks (and other diabetes supplies) puts your child in a position to handle this kind of problem on his own and is consistent with your overall goal of helping him learn to control his own blood sugars. Mom and Dad simply won't be there to do it forever, so it's important for the child to take on this responsibility in age-appropriate steps. The youngest children may simply wear a fanny pack or backpack that was filled by another family member. The next step might be helping choose the specific foods to include. At some point, the child can become part of the kitchen brigade, helping with the actual food preparation. And finally, the child can plan, prepare, and tote his own snacks, touching base with Mom and Dad on occasion to check out the details.

For children who develop diabetes at a very young age, it seems to work quite well to make them responsible for carrying their own snacks from the start. Most toddlers and preschoolers enjoy having their own colorful backpack, fanny pack, or decorated lunch bag (they can decorate the paper ones themselves). They'll probably get in the habit of carrying one if it is presented matter-of-factly. Of course, it's a good idea for Mom and Dad to carry or stash a back-up supply for emergencies, at least in the early years.

Older kids can keep snacks (along with their other diabetes supplies like insulin and blood testing equipment) in the same kinds of book bags, gym bags, and fanny packs that their friends use. There's no reason why diabetes supplies have to look like diabetes supplies when they leave home.

Many parents we've worked with have taken the very wise step of routinely including enough snack food for a friend or friends when preparing or providing snacks. This puts the snacking in a much more positive light; it becomes an opportunity to share with friends rather than a requirement to do something that sets your child apart as different.

What if, in spite of all your support and low-key encouragement, your child consistently refuses or "forgets" (a less assertive form of refusal) to carry snacks or other diabetes needs? Clearly, the safety issues demand that you play backstop for your child. Insulin, food, and blood-testing supplies need to be handy. Use questioning, experimentation, and problem-solving, as described in Chapter 5, to develop mutually acceptable solutions. Address specific situations one at a time. Another option is described in Chapter 14. There, you'll see some examples of how diabetes tasks can be broken down into many separate steps. Even though your child may not be willing to take on complete responsibility for carrying snacks or supplies at this time, you may be able to agree on some small steps toward that eventual goal to get you started. Good luck!

WHAT IF HE SIMPLY WON'T EAT A SNACK?

Children will sometimes just refuse to eat a snack. This refusal can be direct ("I'm not going to eat it!") or indirect (snack foods found in the bottom of the wastebasket after school). Giving the child who balks at the regimen a chance to refuse a snack can defuse a situation. It's also consistent with your respective job descriptions: you provide it, he decides whether or not to eat it. There are several possible outcomes. The child may have no ill effects at all from skipping the snack. This is most likely if his blood sugar was running high to start with. If his blood sugar was fairly normal, the child may start to get mildly low and have a change of heart, finding his missing appetite in a hurry. Or if the blood sugar was on the low side to begin with, the child may go even lower and really need treatment.

That's okay, especially if you're in a controlled setting: home, for example. Remember, people learn from their experiences. It is responsible to allow children to learn the consequences of their diabetes-related behaviors firsthand, in a safe environment. If you let this happen at home without a lot of angst, the child can learn for himself why snacks are important. It's important not to "reinforce" this lesson with a lot of "I told you so's." This may put the child on the defensive, which would detract from any learning that has taken place.

Your judgment in this kind of situation is very important. The same approach would not be a good idea if you knew your kid was heading off on a long bike ride or was set to compete in a sports event. That would remove the situation from a controlled, safe environment. Those kinds of circumstances call for the kind of family problem-solving described in Chapter 5. With that approach, you and your child can work together to find a way for him to get what he wants—to go for the bike ride or compete in the sport event—while you get what you want—for your child to be safe during these activities.

If you have thought of snacks as a burdensome part of your child's care in the past, we hope we have given you a new perspective. Snacks are natural to small children anyway. They smooth out blood sugar control, helping to prevent both after-meal highs and between-meal lows. And perhaps most importantly, they can free you from rigid meal-by-meal plans. Using the time block method can keep food and insulin in sync in spite of your kid's variable appetite and personal quirks.

THE BOTTOM LINE

For All Kids

1. All small children need snacks because of high energy needs and small stomach capacities.

For Kids With Diabetes

1. Snacks help prevent low blood sugar between meals and overnight.
2. Snacks help prevent high blood sugar by spreading food more evenly throughout the day.
3. Snacks containing carbohydrate, protein, and fat do the best job of stabilizing blood sugar control and controlling appetite.
4. Food from meals and snacks in the same insulin time block can be moved around to meet appetite and blood sugar control needs.
5. Include protein, fat, or "Lente carbohydrate" in bedtime snacks to support blood glucose throughout the night.

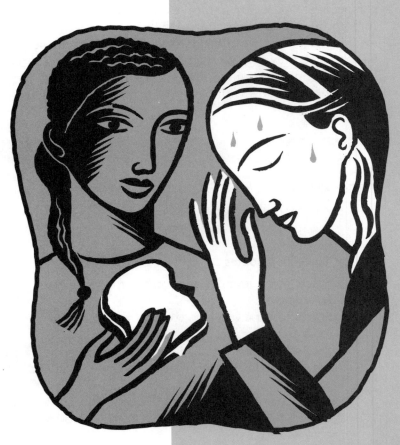

"I could feel myself getting lower and lower,
but I didn't have anything to eat with me..."

Preventing and Treating Low Blood Sugar

Eating a moldy cheese sandwich convinced Lindy that it was a good idea to carry her own food supply.

Lindy was 17 and totally against doing anything that, as she said, "exposed" her diabetes in front of her friends. She refused to add a lunchtime shot to her insulin regimen because she'd have to take it at school. She spent her own money to get the smallest blood sugar meter she could find. She kept it at the bottom of her book bag and only used it (in a bathroom stall) if she was feeling really bad. And her educator's suggestions about carrying snack food to treat low blood sugars were about as welcome as ants at a picnic. Lindy insisted she would be fine because she always carried money to buy a soft drink or candy if she needed to.

With this mind-set, Lindy's educator was quite surprised when she showed up one day for her appointment with a hefty supply of crackers, candy, and some boxed juice in her book bag. What had changed her mind, she wanted to know. Lindy laughed a bit when she explained how she and a friend had been trapped in an elevator at school for nearly 2 hours a few days earlier. The elevator clunked to a stop just before lunch. As the lunch hour ticked by, Lindy could feel her blood sugar getting lower and lower. And, of course, the change she carried to buy food wasn't doing her a bit of good in that elevator. After trying to hide the situation for a while, she finally told her friend what was happening and asked if she had anything to eat with her.

"Sure. I've still got my lunch from a couple of days ago. You're welcome to it." Eating a moldy cheese sandwich convinced Lindy, in a way no amount of advice had been able to, that it was a good idea to carry her own food supply.

Lindy was hardly alone in her problems with low blood sugar. It's not unusual for a child with diabetes to have an average of one low blood sugar episode a week. Fortunately, most of these will be fairly mild, but even the mildest low is unpleasant. More severe episodes can be embarrassing, scary, and even dangerous.

You may also know low blood sugar by the terms "insulin reaction," "hypo," or simply "reaction." But by any name, it means the same thing: trouble.

Hypoglycemia can interfere with your child's thinking, making mental tasks—like doing schoolwork or even getting the food she needs to treat herself—difficult or impossible. Being low can also make physical tasks, such as riding a bicycle or driving a car, hazardous. In addition, if you or your child is really afraid of lows, you or she might intentionally let her blood sugars run high all the time to protect against a low and, in that way, increase her risk for the long-term complications of diabetes. It's not surprising that low blood sugar is a big deal for both of you.

In fact, many parents tell us that hypoglycemia (both the reality and the fear of it) has an extremely powerful negative effect on their family relationships. Arguments arise when parents push their kids to be responsible—to carry food, wear a medical alert identification, and let people know how to respond if they get low and aren't able to treat themselves. Kids, for their part, often vigorously resist all these sensible precautions.

LOW BLOOD SUGAR DEFINED

What exactly do we mean by hypoglycemia? Some people define lows solely by blood glucose level, such as less than 60 mg/dl, but we don't. Just the number isn't enough, because some people do fine with a blood sugar of 60 mg/dl, while others clearly feel hypoglycemic at 80 mg/dl. We think it makes more sense to say that your child is hypoglycemic when her blood sugar is low enough to cause her to feel or act hypoglycemic (more on this in a moment) and she gets over her symptoms when her sugar level comes back up. To help you understand why this type of definition is necessary, let's describe some of the many symptoms that hypoglycemia can cause and how they relate (or don't relate) to the actual blood sugar level.

SYMPTOMS OF HYPOGLYCEMIA

The common symptoms of hypoglycemia fall into three categories: physical, mental, and emotional. You've probably observed all three types of symptoms in your child at various times. As you review these symptoms, keep in mind that different people experience symptoms of hypoglycemia at different blood sugar levels. What's more, the same person may have different symptoms on different days: she may feel anxious and sweaty one day when her blood sugar is 80 mg/dl and not have any symptoms at all a few days later at a blood sugar of 40 mg/dl. Before we go on to explain how this can happen, let's first describe the symptoms we're talking about.

Physical symptoms. Physical symptoms of low blood sugar include trembling, light-headedness or dizziness, pounding heart, and poor coordination. These symptoms are caused by the body trying to protect itself by releasing counterregulatory hormones. These hormones raise your child's blood sugar level by helping the body release stored sugar into the bloodstream. The term counterregulatory refers to the fact that these hormones work opposite to insulin. Insulin lowers blood sugar. These hormones—epinephrine (also called adrenaline), glucagon, cortisol, and growth hormone—raise it. Whenever your child's sugar level falls to a certain point (usually, but not always, about 50 mg/dl), the body releases these counterregulatory hormones.

Adrenaline is the same hormone your child's body releases when she is in any stressful situation. You may have heard of the fight-or-flight response. The physical symptoms of low blood sugar—shaking, trembling, a rapid heart beat, feeling anxious—and those of the fight-or-flight stress response are identical. Even though symptoms such as trembling, sweating, and a pounding heart may be reliable signs that your child is hypoglycemic, they are not a direct result of low blood sugar. Instead, they are the result of her body's efforts to counteract the hypoglycemia.

Other symptoms you might notice when your child is low include visual disturbances (double vision, seeing spots, even temporary partial blindness), sudden hunger, a headache, a stomachache, or sudden and severe fatigue. Some kids tell us one or more of these symptoms are the most reliable sign that they are low. In fact, we are amazed at the variety of symptoms children describe: one will tell us she feels a numbness in her hands; yet another has a feeling that everyone around is moving farther and farther away. Many can't provide any more exact description of how they feel than to say they feel funny.

Mental symptoms. If your child's blood sugar level goes really low, her brain is starved for glucose—the only type of fuel it can use—and it begins to malfunction. In this state, your child is not firing on all cylinders. The mental symptoms of low blood sugar include having difficulty concentrating, being clumsy, spacey, dizzy, or confused, having a headache, speaking with a slur or more slowly than usual, and being tired. *If your child shows any of these signs of moderate to severe hypoglycemia, immediate action is a must.* These signs can indicate that the blood sugar is getting low enough to lead to loss of consciousness or a seizure.

Emotional symptoms. You've probably noticed that low blood sugar can affect your child's mood, too. When she is hypoglycemic she may get irritable, or she may act funny. Parents often pick up on hypoglycemia by subtle (or not so subtle) changes in mood or personality. One father we know gently suggests that his son test his blood sugar whenever he suspects the child is low. If his son reacts angrily with a statement like "Leave me alone. I don't need to test my blood sugar!," Dad tells him, "You're absolutely right, you don't need to test. You can go straight to the orange juice." Since the boy is usually easygoing, his dad has learned that the most likely cause for an angry outburst is hypoglycemia.

LEVELS OF HYPOGLYCEMIA

Despite the wide variations in symptoms and the fact that they are not perfectly reliable, it is worth briefly mentioning those symptoms that are most typical of various levels of hypoglycemia.

Mild hypoglycemia. When your child has mild hypoglycemia, she has the physical and emotional symptoms we identified above in a form that does not interfere significantly with her normal activities. You or she may notice a change in her thought processes, but she doesn't act in a way that is noticeably abnormal to people who don't know her that well. These episodes may be uncomfortable or upsetting, but most often they are only a nuisance and respond quickly to treatment.

Moderate hypoglycemia. With moderate hypoglycemia, there is a more obvious problem, in the form of confusion, inappropriate behavior, or both. But your child is still alert enough to treat her own low blood sugar or to let you know that she needs help. Recovery after treatment typically takes a bit longer compared with mild hypoglycemia.

Severe hypoglycemia. When hypoglycemia is severe, your child is so confused that she cannot self-treat or get help. She may even have a seizure or fall into a coma. If your child has ever had such an episode, you know how terribly upsetting severe hypoglycemia can be. In our experience, these episodes are even harder on parents than they are on kids, since the child is often unconscious and unaware of the seriousness of the situation. A child will usually feel bad for quite some time after a severe low sugar reaction, even after the blood sugar is back to normal.

PROBLEMS WITH SYMPTOMS AS A GUIDE TO BLOOD SUGAR LEVELS

Unfortunately, using symptoms to identify hypoglycemia isn't 100% accurate. First of all, as we've said, different people have different symptoms of low blood sugar. The clues that your child is hypoglycemic may be completely different from another child's clues. Some of your child's symptoms may even be unique. One of us was working with a 7-year-old child who had lots of problems with hypoglycemia. A big difficulty was that he didn't seem to have any of the common symptoms to warn him he was getting low. Then one day the boy joyously reported that he had finally discovered a reliable sign: he got a tickle in the back of his throat. He might be the only person who ever had this symptom, but it worked for him, and that was all that mattered.

You may also notice times that your child feels hypoglycemic when she is not actually low. This could be a case of her trying to talk herself (or you) into believing she needs something to eat. But it could also be the result of her blood sugar coming down very rapidly from a high level, yet still not being low. The body seems to take a rapid drop in blood sugar as a sign of developing hypoglycemia, and it responds by releasing counterregulatory hormones as a protective measure. There also may be times when your child is simply anxious and confuses the symptoms of anxiety with those of hypoglycemia. Furthermore, some children can't feel any real difference between their symptoms of low blood sugar and those they get when their blood sugar is high.

Relying on symptoms is also tricky because your child's hypoglycemic symptoms may vary over time, even from day to day. Sometimes they even disappear almost completely. If your child doesn't feel low until her blood sugar level is well below 50 mg/dl, waiting for symptoms can mean that she will be in serious trouble before she or you can do anything about it.

A child who repeatedly feels no obvious symptoms when the blood sugar is less than 50 mg/dl actually has quite a serious problem. She has lost the early physical warning signs that her blood sugar is dropping dangerously low. This state, called hypoglycemia unawareness, can develop if your child has several episodes of low blood sugar in a short period of time. It happens because the body adapts to frequent lows by becoming better at getting along on smaller and smaller amounts of blood sugar. This adaptation keeps the body from releasing counterregulatory hormones at moderately low blood sugar levels. And there goes the hypoglycemia early-warning system. This is nearly always a temporary situation in children. As you know or can imagine, even this temporary form of hypoglycemia unawareness can be quite a problem because it makes it harder to recognize and treat lows before they become serious. The best way to restore normal early-warning symptoms is to avoid all hypoglycemia for a few days.

For all the shortcomings of symptoms, however, recognizing them is still a major key to avoiding serious problems. Both you and your child need to be on the alert for her own particular symptoms. When watchfulness is coupled with frequent and timely blood sugar testing, you will identify many developing lows before they get serious.

CAUSES AND PREVENTION OF HYPOGLYCEMIA

When your child's blood sugar is low, the culprit is almost always one or more of the following things: near-normal control, too much insulin, too little food, or too much exercise. Older youngsters can also have low blood sugar problems because of drinking alcohol or, in girls, because of the hormonal changes of the menstrual cycle.

Near-normal control. Working hard, with intensive regimens, to keep your child's blood sugars as close to normal as possible increases her risk of hypoglycemia. That's because there's much less margin for error if you are aiming for near-normal levels than there is if blood sugar is staying higher. As we discussed previously, the DCCT intensive treatment group had three times as much hypoglycemia as participants in the trial who practiced conventional treatment.

Since the risk of hypoglycemia goes up a lot when you try for tight blood sugar control, you and your child have to work hard to anticipate and prevent problems. We know it's impossible to do this all the time, and getting your child to cooperate can be a major challenge, but there are some guidelines to keep in mind. First, be aware of the near-lows. If your child always tends to run 70 to 90 mg/dl at some particular time during the day or night, once in a while her blood sugar will be 50 mg/dl, and she will be in trouble. Try not to cut it too close. A bit less insulin or a bit more food can correct a pattern of near-lows, reducing risk for hypoglycemia.

Next, ease up a little on glucose goals when the situation calls for it. If your child has been having lots of lows, for example, don't push so hard to keep her blood sugars down, at least for a few days. As we've mentioned, a vicious cycle can start: low blood sugars reduce her ability to detect low blood sugars, so having lots of lows can make for more lows. Remember, even a few days free from hypoglycemia can restore the ability to detect low blood sugar symptoms. Frequent lows—especially if they're severe—can deplete the body's supplies of stored sugar. If this happens, the body can no longer protect itself against serious lows because an important safety net has been lost. Eating enough food, taking enough insulin, and avoiding severe lows allows the body to rebuild its stores of sugar.

You may also want to ease up for specific situations in which low blood sugar would be a real problem: an athletic event, driving a car, or a camping trip, for instance. This can be a tricky business, of course, since these same stressful situations could push her blood sugars higher anyway. And, of course, being high creates its own acute problems.

Finally, you may need to adjust your goals for glycemic control if your child is younger than 7 years of age. This is important for two reasons. First, in the first few years of life, your child's brain is still developing, and she needs glucose for this purpose. Low blood sugars during this period can hurt her by interfering with brain and nervous system development. Second, a very young child may be less able than an older child to let you know when she is getting hypoglycemic. You may not be able to distinguish the signs of low blood sugar from normal fussiness or sleepiness. When a very young child is low and you don't know it, you may not be able to treat her hypoglycemia in a timely manner.

Too much insulin. Taking too much insulin before breakfast contributes to daytime episodes of hypoglycemia. Too much morning Regular insulin can make your child low from about mid-morning to before lunch. And too much morning NPH or Lente insulin can make her low anytime from about lunchtime until before dinner. Early morning (1 to 3 A.M.) hypoglycemia, caused by too much NPH or Lente insulin at dinner or bedtime, is also fairly common.

Hypoglycemia can also be caused by uneven or changed absorption of insulin. Uneven absorption is a characteristic of injected insulin and is pretty much uncontrollable. Ultralente insulin tends to be more variable than Lente. Lente is more unpredictable than NPH. NPH is more variable than Regular insulin. Changed absorption of insulin, on the other hand, is sometimes caused by exercise, something you and your child do have control over. If your child exercises a part of her body into which she has just injected insulin (such as running after injecting into the thigh), faster insulin absorption may trigger low blood sugar. Absorption can also be speeded up by heat (such as a hot tub, warm bath, shower, or even laying in the sun at the beach), bringing on low blood sugar because the insulin peaks earlier than usual.

We've also seen lows happen when people started a new bottle of insulin. This can happen because insulin slowly loses its strength once the vial is started. If a bottle lasts a very long time (as it does in kids who take tiny insulin doses), the insulin may weaken quite a bit. Insulin doses may get progressively increased to make up for the loss of strength. Taking the same dose from a new, full-strength vial of insulin will then push the blood sugar too low. Also, if your child switches to a more purified insulin, or from mixed species to single species, or to human insulin, her blood sugars may dip if the same doses are used. Anytime you switch insulins, it's a good idea to do more frequent blood testing so that any needed dose changes can be made as quickly as possible.

When your child has several episodes of low blood sugar in a row at the same time of day, you'll have to cut down her dose on your own or with the help of your health-care provider. Since your goal is to help your child learn to control her own blood sugars, talk through the reasoning behind any changes with the child. Even children too young to make such decisions on their own can begin to absorb the reasons and techniques. Being included in the process will build her confidence and competence for managing when she's on her own.

The presence of a certain amount of extra insulin between meals and overnight can't be avoided with most of the insulins we have available (Regular, NPH, Lente, and Ultralente). It's just the way these insulin formulations are absorbed and used by the body. (Figure 6.1 compares the action of injected insulins to the body's own insulin.) But there are a couple of tools that can help produce insulin levels that are more like the body's own.

One tool that can reduce excess insulin is the insulin pump. Pumps meter out insulin in small, precise amounts throughout the day and night. This reduces the risk for hypoglycemia. But, for a variety of reasons, pumps aren't used very much for younger kids. For one thing, they're expensive. Health insurance often covers the cost, but for a family without coverage, finances can be a barrier. Probably the biggest reason that pumps don't get recommended a lot for youngsters, however, is that very few health-care providers have experience using them. There are a few pediatric diabetes programs around the country that have great success using pumps in teens and in kids as young as 10. Unfortunately, these centers are the exception rather than the rule. Doctors without that experience are less likely to recommend a pump. If there is a diabetes team in your area that has skill and experience with pumps, it might be worth considering—both for the pump's ability to lower hypoglycemia risk and for the greater flexibility for meals and exercise that it provides.

Another promising possibility for reducing hypoglycemia risk is a totally new insulin called Humalog (Eli Lilly and Company). It will be coming on the market throughout the world during 1996 and 1997. Compared with our current insulins, it has some very small changes in its chemical makeup that make it act faster than Regular insulin and very much like the body's own meal-related doses of insulin. It comes on very quickly and then disappears quickly as well, reducing the risk for low blood sugars between meals. Some of its other advantages over Regular insulin are listed in Table 7.1. Humalog certainly won't totally eliminate low blood sugar as a concern, but it definitely will be a better tool for some kids in helping cut the risk.

Too little food. Skipping meals or snacks, delaying them more than 30 to 60 minutes, or eating less food or less carbohydrate than usual can lead to low blood sugars. This is less likely if the premeal blood sugar level is high.

This is, of course, why parents can be driven to distraction when their child takes her premeal insulin and then refuses to eat. Visions of severe low blood sugar and calls to 911 lead them to begin frantically (and often angrily) pressuring the child to eat. The result is never pretty, and it usually doesn't work. As we discussed earlier, pressuring almost always results in kids actually eating less, not more. What can you do if you find yourself in this pickle? If at all possible, we'd like to prevent these situations, but if you find yourself with a balky child full of insulin, it's no time to think about what you should have done to prevent it. Instead, we

TABLE 7.1 Facts About Humalog (Eli Lilly and Company), New Mealtime Insulin

- A rapidly absorbed version of human insulin with an action profile similar to the way the body puts out insulin during a meal.

- Used with meals in place of Regular insulin. NPH, Lente, or Ultralente insulin must be used with Humalog to meet basal (between meals and overnight) insulin needs.

- Doses are, unit for unit, like Regular insulin.

- Begins to work almost immediately; peaks in about an hour; lasts only about 3 hours.

- May help reduce the risk of hypoglycemia between meals because of its shorter period of action.

- Provides excellent control of after-meal blood sugars when taken with the meal. When Regular insulin is taken with the meal, after-meal blood sugars tend to be elevated.

- No need to remember or make time for a test and injection 30 to 45 minutes before eating. All care can be done right at mealtime.

recommend you let your child eat anything healthy that suits her and will supply the amount of carbohydrate that's in the usual meal.

For example, Mom gives 5-year-old Johnny his usual five units of Regular insulin to cover his usual evening meal containing about 75 grams of carbohydrate (3 Starch, 1 Milk, 1 Vegetable, and 1 Fruit). But Johnny played hard this afternoon. Tired and cranky, he takes one look at the tuna-noodle casserole that's for dinner and starts to cry. "That's yucky," he wails. "I don't want any." Since his blood sugar was 97 mg/dl before supper, Mom knows he's going to need something pretty soon to cover the insulin. Being a wise woman, she avoids getting into a shouting match over the casserole. "I'm sorry you don't like what we're having, Johnny, but since you already took your insulin and you played so hard this afternoon, you need to eat something. We've got some other things on the table that you like. What looks good to you?"

Johnny may choose the bread that's on the table for dinner. Mom can throw in some peanut butter to sweeten the pot, if that will increase the likelihood of the bread being eaten. With milk and fruit, it should be possible to replace the 75 grams of carbohydrate without too much fuss.

If the child's appetite is really poor, offer more concentrated sources of carbohydrate so you cover the insulin with less total food volume. For example, this is no time to offer the reduced-calorie cranberry juice cocktail (1 cup = 15 grams of carbohydrate). Instead, go for grape juice or a fruit nectar (1/3 cup = 15 grams of carbohydrate). Skip the popcorn (3 cups in a 15-gram carbohydrate portion) and go directly to a biscuit or a muffin (1 small muffin = 15 grams of carbohydrate). The best choices will, of course, depend on your child's preferences, but you get the idea. When appetite or food acceptance are poor, offer choices that are both well-liked and fairly concentrated. Do your very best to avoid pressuring the child to eat. It's counterproductive. Also try to avoid offering sweets only at times like this. It might encourage the child to act up in order to get things that aren't usually available. (See Chapter 5 for tips on incorporating sweets into meals.) And remember, the sugar in chocolate and other candies that contain a lot of fat may be absorbed more slowly, so they might not be the best choices for times like this. However, what works best to raise low blood glucose is quite individual. If one thing doesn't work, try another. One 2-year-old child we know refused to eat or drink anything when she was low. Her mom finally discovered that if she just set three candy-coated chocolate drops in front of the little girl, without trying to get her to eat them, the child would slowly and cautiously stick one in her mouth. This actually raised her blood sugar enough that Mom could get a little cooperation in drinking some juice. Creativity and an open mind can work wonders.

Also keep in mind that most of the insulins we use (Regular, NPH, Lente, and Ultralente) have very long activity periods, compared with the body's own insulin. Because of this, you can take some of the pressure off of feeling your child has to eat exactly the right amount at every meal and snack. If dinner is on the light side, add that missing carbohydrate to the next snack. If you think that acceptance may still be a problem, offer it in a form (preferred and concentrated, as described above) that makes it more likely to be eaten. Say Johnny only ate 60 grams of carbohydrate (compared with his usual 75-gram supper) after the big tuna-noodle casserole fiasco. Mom could easily add the other 15 grams of carbohydrate to his usual 30-gram carbohydrate bedtime snack by substituting a cup of fruit juice for his usual cup of milk: same total volume of food to eat, but more concentrated in carbohydrate. This will work fine since he'll get the same 105 grams of carbohydrate during the time his Regular insulin is working as if he had eaten the usual meal and snack. (Refer to Chapter 6 for more information about how moving food between a meal and a snack can help you deal with variations in your child's appetite.)

Kids don't willingly starve themselves.

● ● ● ●

If this mealtime dilemma happens a lot, another option to consider is that of delaying the insulin until after your child has eaten. This tactic is not uncommon with infants, toddlers, and preschoolers whose intake may be quite unpredictable or who go on food jags. Taking insulin after the meal is not the greatest idea in terms of blood sugar control, but it's a lot better than turning dinnertime into a donnybrook. The Humalog insulin analog will be a better insulin for this type of use, since its onset is so rapid that you apparently can get quite good blood sugar control taking it immediately after a meal.

Yet another way to reduce hypoglycemia risk in little kids on an "I'm not going to eat" tear is to reduce by half the insulin dose that covers the problem mealtime. Try this for a few days. With so much less insulin around you can feel relaxed about letting her eat as little as she wants. This can break the cycle and allow you to readjust insulin as food intake stabilizes.

We think that once you find a way to prevent your child's food refusal from becoming a scene, she will probably stop refusing in fairly short order. Remember, kids don't willingly starve themselves. They generally only get really balky about food over long periods of time if we turn it into a battle of wills by trying to force the issue

Too much activity. Speaking of the ways kids' lifestyles can contradict efforts to minimize the risk of low blood sugars, consider the difficulties of managing unplanned, prolonged, or high-intensity physical activity. And what child doesn't play this way? Activity can cause a child's blood sugars to drop like a stone. We know children who come home from a day sitting around at school with a blood sugar of 240 mg/dl, play actively for 30 to 45 minutes, and end up with a blood sugar reading of 80 mg/dl. We talk more about exercise in Chapter 8, where we discuss, among other things, the fact that the hypoglycemic effect of exercise can be immediate or delayed. It may last for as long as 24 hours.

Though it's much easier said than done, it's best if your child tests her blood anytime she's planning to exercise. That way, if the result suggests there's a reasonable chance she will go low during her activity, she can eat something before she starts. In addition, she should always have a source of fast-acting carbohydrate available when she exercises, in case she begins to go low. We talk more later in this chapter about ways to help your child learn to take these essential precautions.

Drinking alcohol. If your child drinks alcoholic beverages (even as little as 2 to 3 ounces of alcohol), it can suppress glucose release from the liver and increase her risk of hypoglycemia. When her blood sugar is low and she has been drinking, her liver loses its usual ability to pour glucose into the blood, leaving her without a vital safety net to protect her from dangerously low blood sugar.

This may be an almost impossible topic to discuss with your child, since she's unlikely to talk about it openly with you. Yet it's so important that you try, if you even suspect she might be drinking. Approach her without judgment (if you can), and simply share the facts with her, or ask her diabetes health-care provider to raise the issue.

Your child needs to know that if she's planning to drink alcohol, she should have something to eat first. That way she won't be depending on the glucose reserves in her liver to protect her from hypoglycemia. She needs to understand she's dependent on the food she eats to protect her from going low. She also needs to know that hypoglycemia can easily be mistaken for drunken behavior. The friends she's with should know about her diabetes, and she should be carrying or wearing some form of diabetes identification. Hopefully she will never drink to excess—it's just too much of a risk with diabetes—but if she does, these precautions will help protect her from a bad outcome.

Menstrual cycle. Some young women tell us that their insulin requirements go down dramatically each time their periods begin. This often follows a few days of increased insulin needs just before the onset of menses. The pattern is caused by shifting hormone levels. If your daughter has increased her insulin doses to deal with rising blood sugars before her period begins, she may become hypoglycemic as her insulin needs go back down after the flow starts.

If your daughter tends to have blood sugar fluctuations related to her menstrual cycle, she should keep really close track of the pattern. This will allow her to figure out how to raise and lower her insulin doses at the earliest possible moment in order to avoid extremes of hyperglycemia just before her period and hypoglycemia once her flow starts.

TREATING HYPOGLYCEMIA

No matter how hard you try, you can't prevent all of your child's low blood sugars. You both need to be prepared to deal with the low blood sugars that do occur. Since we don't know how old your child is, or whether you will be there to help deal with her hypoglycemia, we offer the following suggestions assuming that you are there. If you're not, your child or another responsible person will have to manage the situation. It's your job to help your child learn to deal with those low blood sugars she's capable of managing on her own. It's also your responsibility to see to it that those adults who spend a significant amount of time with your child (teachers, coaches, grandparents, her friend's parents, youth group leaders, and others) know what they need to do if your child has low blood sugar while she is with them.

Treat immediately. If you test and find your child's blood sugar is low, or if you can't test but you suspect she's low based on how she feels or how she's acting, get her something to eat or drink right away. All too often children ignore the early warning signs of low blood sugar. They tell themselves they can hold out another 10, 30, or even 60 minutes. Kids generally hate to acknowledge that they are low (it's embarrassing). They also hate to stop what they are doing. Unfortunately, delaying treatment can only lead to more severe low blood sugar.

Plan ahead. Have glucose tablets or other appropriate carbohydrates in your pocket or purse, in your car, or anywhere else where you may be with your child. And encourage her to do the same. It's our impression that this works best if it's made the child's responsibility from the youngest possible age (not that Mom and Dad don't also carry or stash backup supplies). Even very young kids can carry fanny packs or colorful lunch or snack bags, or have supplies in a book bag or backpack. However, as the story we told about Lindy at the beginning of the chapter suggests, this doesn't always work, especially with youngsters who are hesitant about revealing their diabetes to others. In fact, one of the most common frustrations we hear from parents of kids with diabetes is that their child will not carry food to prevent and treat low blood sugars. Sometimes this changes when the child has a scary or unpleasant experience, as Lindy did. After all, we all learn best from our own experience.

You may also be able to help your child by problem-solving for an approach that she might find acceptable. Remember all the suggestions we made in Chapter 5, where we talked about helping your child learn to manage her own diabetes? She has effective veto power, so pushing her will not work, as you know all too well. The key is working with her to learn what would motivate her to carry the needed supplies. Then continue to work together to find mutually acceptable ways to keep her safe. Make it clear to her from the outset that any suggestion you offer is off the table if she doesn't like it. That way she might not block you out, and you might get somewhere in your efforts to help her learn how to stay safe.

Specifics of Hypoglycemia Treatment

Mild hypoglycemia. Mild, and even some moderate, hypoglycemia can be treated with 10 to 15 grams of fast-acting carbohydrate. Some examples are

- 2 or 3 glucose tablets (5 grams each)
- 1/3 to 1/2 of 30-gram tube of glucose gel
- 1/3 to 1/2 of a small tube of cake frosting
- 3 to 4 ounces of orange juice
- 4 to 6 ounces of regular soda
- 1/4 to 1/3 cup of raisins
- 5 Lifesavers candies
- 1 cup of milk
- Any high-carbohydrate, low-fat food that your child likes

If you're tempted to treat with much more food than these amounts, don't do it—at least initially. Giving more does not speed up recovery, and it may send blood sugar shooting way back up.

Repeat this treatment in 15 to 30 minutes if your child's low blood sugar symptoms continue or if her blood sugar level is still below 60 mg/dl. The exact amount of these foods that will work best for your child depends to some extent on her body size and on exactly how low the blood sugar is to begin with. The smaller the body, the more rise of blood sugar that's produced by a given amount of carbohydrate. If you find that your child's blood sugars are consistently bouncing back too high after treating low blood sugar, you might try cutting the size of the carbohydrate portion you're using.

Remember, high-fat sweets like chocolate and ice cream are not good treatment choices for most kids because the fat can slow down absorption of the sugar they contain.

If the next meal or snack is more than an hour away, you need to follow up the initial treatment of any low blood sugar with an additional carbohydrate snack that also provides protein and fat. The easily absorbed carbohydrates that bring blood sugar up quickly don't last for very long—probably not more than an hour. That's why a more substantial and slowly digested snack is needed. Crackers and cheese, a peanut butter sandwich (whole, half, or quarter, depending on the child's size and on how far away the next meal or snack is), or a similar snack will protect your child from a recurrence of the low blood sugar.

Moderate hypoglycemia. Moderate hypoglycemia usually can be treated in the same way as mild low blood sugar, though it may take more than one treatment, and it may take longer to fully recover. The stronger the symptoms—confusion, clumsiness, slurred speech, headache, and so on—the slower the recovery. Where a child may feel perfectly fine within a few minutes after treating a very mild reaction, it may take 30 to 45 minutes to feel totally normal again following a moderate reaction. It's at times like these that many people overtreat their low blood sugars. This is understandable. After all, the symptoms are uncomfortable, to put it mildly. If you're feeling shaky, confused, ravenously hungry, and anxious, with your heart beating rapidly, you want all those feelings to just go away! People tend to eat and drink until the symptoms are gone. It's hard to remember at times like these that it's the first 15 or 30 grams of carbohydrate that do the trick. One of our patients described his treatment for those stronger lows like this: "I just empty out the refrigerator until I feel better. Last time it was about a quart of orange juice, two or three slices of bread, and half of a Snickers bar. My next blood sugar was almost 400."

This tendency to overtreat is particularly strong in children and adults who have had previous bad experiences with hypoglycemic episodes. Kids may have the additional motivation of wanting to get back immediately to whatever they were doing before they became hypoglycemic. Kids are also somewhat less likely than adults to have the restraint required to consume only the amount of food they need to get their blood sugar level back to normal. And parents can feel so panicked by their child's hypoglycemia that they, also, have the tendency to treat very aggressively in hopes that the child will feel better that much sooner.

Natural as the tendency might be to treat your child's hypoglycemia until she feels better, by the time you are done treating, her blood sugar is probably well on its way to being sky high. You might be able to curb this tendency if you use commercially prepared glucose tablets and gels to treat her hypoglycemia. These products are premeasured and not overly yummy, so you are less likely to overuse them. If your child simply can't stand these products, you might try preparing a low blood sugar first-aid package, containing just enough food (15 to 30 grams of carbohydrate) to rescue her from most low blood sugar emergencies.

Finally, you might use the approach (and try to teach your child the approach) one of our patients came up with. She made up a little ditty that she repeated to herself as she waited for the food she had eaten to bring her blood sugar back up. It went something like this: "Relax, you'll be fine. You can wait a little, you'll be fine." The key, she said, was to keep the message reassuring and simple. Keep reminding yourself that you are doing the right thing and that everything will be all right. Hard as it might be to believe this when your child is in the throes of a low blood sugar reaction, what you are saying to yourself is true. Try your best to stay calm and confident.

Severe hypoglycemia. When your child is severely hypoglycemic, by definition, she cannot treat herself. She cannot even ask for help. It is essential that you or anyone else your child might be with at the time knows what to do. It is very important that you and these people know not to put anything in her mouth unless she is sitting up and able to swallow. We have seen tragic consequences when a family member tried to pour something sweet into the mouth of a semiconscious youngster. Usually, even with severe hypoglycemia, a person can be coaxed into eating or drinking something sweet. If this is possible, stick with small sips of liquid, or try bits of honey, frosting, or glucose gel placed or rubbed between the cheek and gum. Avoid anything that needs chewing, because the coordination will not be there to do it. If you can't coax a bit of cooperation out of the child, don't force anything into the mouth. Immediately inject glucagon or, if none is available, call 911.

Glucagon Emergency Kit

As we have already mentioned, glucagon is a natural counterregulatory hormone. It is available by prescription in a Glucagon Emergency Kit. The kit contains dry crystals of glucagon and a syringe full of liquid. When it is mixed and injected, it will cause your child's liver to release glucose into her bloodstream and raise her blood sugar level. Glucagon is the best treatment for severe hypoglycemia because it can be used immediately—no waiting for a paramedic to arrive, no wild ride to the emergency room. That means the child spends less time at a dangerously low blood sugar level.

Every family needs to have glucagon. If your physician hasn't already suggested keeping glucagon around, we recommend that you ask for a prescription at your next appointment. And if your child has a history of severe hypoglycemia, don't even wait that long. Call now. You and other family members need to know when and how to give it to your child. Your educator or nurse can show you. Be assured that it is a safe drug. You can't give too much, but it's common to give only half of the dose in the kit to infants and toddlers. Because of their small body size, they simply don't need as much to do the job.

Every family needs to have glucagon.

●　●　●　●

Stored in the refrigerator, glucagon is good for several years, but do be aware of the expiration date on your kit. Since you probably won't need it often, be sure to replace it before the expiration date. Periodically review the instructions for administering glucagon with anyone who might need to do it. The instructions are on a sheet in the box containing the glucagon. See Table 7.2 for guidelines for using glucagon.

Medical Alert Identification

Medical alert identification can be a lifesaver. When your child is away from home, a medical I.D. bracelet, necklace, or wallet card will let anyone coming to her aid know that she has diabetes and takes insulin. Unfortunately, many kids strongly resist wearing anything that announces the fact that they have diabetes. If your child is one of them, be sure to offer her all of the choices available (necklace, bracelet, wallet card). Necklaces and bracelets are available in different metals and designs, as well. If she is resisting, work with her to see if you can find a form of identification she will accept.

One teenager we know, Sam, had several bad episodes of low blood sugar, but he refused to wear any of the commercial

TABLE 7.2 Guidelines for Using Glucagon

- It's almost impossible to make a mistake giving glucagon. Inject in any site. Give the whole vial or half of it.

- Make sure the person administering the glucagon knows to call for emergency assistance if your child doesn't respond to treatment within 15 to 30 minutes.

- Your child's stomach is likely to be upset after you have administered the glucagon; she may vomit. Turn her on her side after giving the shot. This will help prevent choking if she does vomit.

- As soon as your child is alert and able to swallow, offer her something light, such as soda or crackers. She must eat to replace the glucose stores that the glucagon has just released.

- As soon as your child is able to hold down food, have her eat something more substantial that contains protein, such as a sandwich or some milk.

- If nausea or vomiting continues, contact your health-care provider.

medical alert products. This drove his parents crazy. One day when he and his dad came to the diabetes clinic, a counselor helped them find a solution. It turned out that Sam was a talented artist and his father a skilled metal worker. The counselor suggested that Sam design a medical alert necklace he would be willing to wear and have his dad make it for him. They both loved the idea, and several months later, Sam returned for his next clinic visit proudly wearing the most awesome medical alert necklace we've ever seen.

There's always a solution, though it's sometimes hard to find. The key to success is working together to meet both your needs and your child's. Sam's dad wanted him to be safe, and Sam wanted to look cool (or at least not look uncool). As long as each of them focused all his energy on pushing his own position, they were stuck. As soon as they collaborated to meet both their needs, they found a wonderful solution.

SPECIAL PROBLEMS IN TREATING HYPOGLYCEMIA

Rebound Hyperglycemia

We've mentioned that counterregulatory hormones raise your child's blood sugar level. This can protect her from becoming severely hypoglycemic. But this protective mechanism can backfire. If the body jumps in with its protection before you or your youngster can jump in with treatment, the body gets a double whammy: all the glucose from the food plus all the glucose released by the counterregulatory hormones. The result can be a truly stratospheric blood sugar a few hours after a hypoglycemic episode.

If your child had a normally functioning pancreas, this wouldn't happen. Your pancreas (if you don't have diabetes), for example, would simply put out some extra insulin to balance the effects of the counterregulatory hormones, preventing the blood sugar from going too high. But because the pancreas doesn't function normally in diabetes, rebound high blood sugar can occur. What's worse, it can set up a roller coaster ride of more insulin, more hypoglycemia, and even more rebound hyperglycemia. To minimize this problem, it's important to catch and treat reactions early, while they are still mild, whenever possible. This generally prevents the body from getting the real danger signals that trigger a further release of counterregulatory hormones. It's also helpful to avoid those "clean out the refrigerator" treatment binges. But what's probably most important is to be very conservative and methodical in how you change insulin doses after a bad hypoglycemic episode. If you can bring those rebound highs down slowly without overcorrecting and causing another low, you've done a great job.

Nighttime Hypoglycemia

Severe low blood sugar reactions happen most often at night. There are several reasons for this. First, most people have their lowest insulin needs of the day (often 20 to 30% lower than at other times) at 2 to 3 A.M. This occurs at the very time that NPH or Lente insulin taken with the evening meal is likely to have its strongest effect (peak). Also, a person is less likely to notice any symptoms of developing hypoglycemia during sleep. This allows low blood sugar to get worse, because treatment isn't given in the early stages.

To avoid nighttime hypoglycemia, always test your child's blood before she goes to bed. If the reading is less than 120 mg/dl (your team may use a different value, so ask), you may want to increase the size or makeup of the bedtime snack to provide better protection against a nighttime low. This is doubly important if she was very active during the day. Since the time you're concerned about is several hours away, just giving more starch or sugar will not necessarily provide protection when it's really needed. You want something that will keep the blood sugar from falling in 4 or 5 hours. The things that seem to accomplish this best are protein and fat or "Lente carbohydrate," starches that are digested and released quite slowly.

For example, 6-year-old Germaine's usual bedtime snack is composed of three graham cracker squares and a glass of milk (27 grams of carbohydrate or 1 Starch and 1 Milk). She goes out roller-skating that afternoon, and when Mom tests her blood at bedtime, it's only 97 mg/dl. To help keep Germaine out of trouble overnight, Mom has a couple of options for increasing the bedtime snack. She could increase the protein and fat by putting peanut butter or ricotta cheese on the graham crackers. Or, she could switch to a "Lente carbohydrate" source like oatmeal or refried beans (at least out West, even little kids like bean burritos!). (Refer to Chapter 6 for more information on bedtime snacks that provide good protection against lows.)

If nighttime low blood sugars are a problem for your child, it may also be a good idea to check her predawn blood sugar levels from time to time. Some health-care providers also recommend switching the evening dose of NPH or Lente insulin from dinnertime to bedtime. While this means an extra shot each day, it dramatically reduces the risk of nighttime hypoglycemia. This is true because intermediate-acting insulin taken at bedtime peaks around the time the child wakes up, rather than several hours earlier. As mentioned previously, another option is to change the predinner NPH or Lente insulin to Ultralente.

GETTING THE JOB DONE WHEN EMOTIONS ARE OUT OF SORTS

You no doubt have noticed how low blood sugar changes your child's behavior. Sometimes these changes are subtle, maybe a little change in voice or talking pattern that only you are aware of. Other times, hypoglycemia may cause your child to become negative, stubborn, irritable, or even verbally or physically abusive. And severe hypoglycemia may even cause her to act totally out of it, vague and disoriented, bumping into furniture, aimlessly picking things up and putting them down, or just sitting and staring into space. You may also notice emotional signs of hypoglycemia: excitement, sadness, or rapid mood swings, for example.

In any of these states, it can be difficult to get your child to do the right things to treat her low blood sugar. She may fight you or simply refuse to cooperate. Like it or not—and you probably don't—you have to be prepared to help manage the situation. Learn to recognize the signs of low blood sugar. Have a plan and the means for setting things right again.

Find a way to deal with your own feelings when this responsibility is thrust upon you. First, try to resist the natural temptation to lash out or to walk away from the whole mess. At the moment, you are the only one with a fairly normally functioning brain, so you need to use it. One mother we know kept her cool by telling herself that the person she was dealing with was not her darling son but his evil hypoglycemic twin, and that her son would reappear magically if she did the right thing and didn't take his behavior personally.

Finally, learn to administer glucagon. We know it's frightening to think of being responsible for giving your child a shot when she is lying there unconscious. The temptation to simply call 911 may be almost overwhelming. But if you can bring yourself to use glucagon, you can provide your child the fastest possible treatment and avoid the trauma and expense of dealing with emergency medical personnel and hospital staff.

Hypoglycemia is awful. We hope what you've learned from this chapter will help you avoid low blood sugars more often and treat them more quickly and effectively when they do occur.

THE BOTTOM LINE

1. Low blood sugar impairs physical and mental functioning. It can also be scary and embarrassing and hurt family relationships.

2. Low blood sugar symptoms vary from person to person and from day to day. You and your child need to recognize her unique symptoms of low blood sugar.

3. Most low blood sugar is caused by near-normal control, too much insulin, too little food, or too much exercise. Most low blood sugar can be prevented by proper planning.

4. Even when you're very careful, low blood sugar will still happen sometimes. That's why you and your child must always be prepared to treat lows.

5. The right treatment given right away stops mild hypoglycemia from becoming more serious.

6. Treat mild and moderate hypoglycemia with 10 to 15 grams of fast-acting carbohydrate. If the next meal is more than an hour away, follow treatment with a substantial snack.

7. Every family needs to have glucagon. If you don't already have it, ask for a prescription and learn how to use it.

8. Medical alert identification can save a life in the event of severe hypoglycemia. Find a form your child will wear or carry.

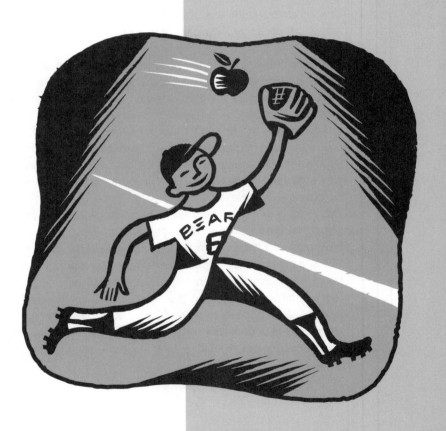

"If Larry eats before baseball practice, he feels sick,
if he doesn't eat, he goes low..."

Managing Sports, Food, and Diabetes

Larry had been running circles around everybody ever since he first climbed out of his crib at the ripe old age of 11 months.

Larry was a really active kid. His parents said he'd been running circles around everybody ever since he first climbed out of his crib on his own at the ripe old age of 11 months. Now that he was in middle school, his whole life revolved around the changing calendar of school and after-school sports. Fall was football season, followed by soccer, baseball, and then summer vacation with camp and swim team.

Larry was 12 the summer his diabetes was diagnosed. The first thing he and his parents asked for was advice about how to manage a coming swim meet. With only 2 weeks to learn the tricks of the trade, they had their work cut out for them. Even though Larry didn't win any ribbons at that first meet, the fact that he swam in two events only 2 weeks after learning he had diabetes was a big victory in itself.

We soon found out at least part of the reason behind Larry's extreme drive to stay active in spite of his diabetes. You see,

Larry was not the first child in the family to develop diabetes. His 14-year-old cousin Jukie had been diagnosed 6 years earlier when she was 8. Larry told us he was determined not to be a couch potato like Jukie. The girl hadn't always been so inactive. But in the early months of dealing with her diabetes, she had a number of fairly severe low blood sugar reactions that had greatly affected her and her parents.

The first time, she passed out while riding her bike and sprained her wrist in the fall. A few weeks later she nearly fainted while playing soccer. The third episode, complete with a seizure, happened during the night following a long hike with her Brownie troop. Jukie's parents decided that it would be easier and safer to keep her still than to have so many low blood sugars. That was when Jukie started spending most of her free time watching TV—a lifestyle Larry had no desire to share.

Whether they are participating in organized sports (like Larry) or just engaging in normal play (like Jukie did before her parents lowered the boom on exercise), most kids have varied levels of physical activity. Managing the changing balance among food, activity, and insulin can be a huge challenge. But it's so important. Handling it well keeps diabetes from being a barrier to normal play or participation in sports. After all, play is truly a child's work, and diabetes shouldn't stand in the way of so basic a need.

Organized sports and other forms of active play are a great way for your child to stay in shape, spend time with friends, build self-confidence, and generally have a lot of fun. Ideally, active play (exercise) should be part of every kid's life; having diabetes makes it even more important. Wonderful as it is, however, playing actively requires your child with diabetes (and you) to plan pretty carefully so that hypoglycemia and other potential problems don't spoil the fun like they did for Jukie.

BENEFITS OF EXERCISE

Since exercise has a dark side for our kids with diabetes (primarily hypoglycemia risk), why should we bother with all the work it takes to make it possible? Because it also has some very important benefits. These benefits fall into three categories: physical, emotional, and social.

Physical Benefits

A fit body. Strength, endurance, coordination, balance: all of these are a direct result of being physically active. Whether it's riding a bike with friends or playing on the all-state basketball team, exercise helps your child have the strong, healthy, flexible body that nature intended. As children move into the preteen and teen years, when appearance becomes more of an issue, the fact that a fit body is also an energetic and attractive body is another big plus.

A stronger, healthier heart. When your child exercises, his muscles work harder and grow stronger. You may not often think about it this way, but his heart is a muscle just like the muscles of his arms or legs. Vigorous exercise builds his heart's capacity to work harder without straining, like lifting weights builds stronger biceps. Exercise also helps keep blood pressure and blood fat levels normal, other important factors in heart health.

Lower blood sugar. You've probably noticed that when your child plays actively for even a short period of time (30 minutes or so), his blood sugar can drop dramatically. Many kids come home after sitting all day at school with a blood sugar reading well into the 200s, go outside to play for awhile, and then come back in complaining of feeling low. Another blood sugar test may reveal that the blood sugar has dropped a lot, even as much as 100 points. Many families use this fact very successfully in controlling blood sugar by sending a child out to play when sugars drift up. Be careful, however, that doing this doesn't make you and your child look at exercise as a punishment for high blood sugars. Try to see it as a side effect of the play and sports your child enjoys: a side effect you can sometimes use to your advantage. As you already know, although this glucose-lowering effect of exercise can be a very good thing, it can also be a challenge to stable blood sugar control. This is especially true if exercise (play) isn't quite regular in both time and amount (and not many children play as long and as hard at the same time every day). There are ways to manage that challenge successfully so your child can enjoy all the benefits of play and sports.

Weight control. Obesity is a large and growing problem among our young people, and lack of exercise is a big factor in that problem. Not that everyone is meant to be thin. Some kids are stocky by nature, others are more average, and a few are naturally thin. But as we've said before, exercise helps normalize the appetite and keep it in tune with the body's real need for calories. Being active is especially helpful to kids who are already carrying around more body fat than is healthy or who have difficulty maintaining a healthy weight. It helps these kids achieve and maintain their own best weight without cutting way back on the food they eat. Actually, aggressive dieting and weight loss are not recommended for kids who are still growing. Rather, helping even quite heavy youngsters stop or minimize weight gain through a combination of exercise and better food choices is a more effective and responsible road to take. This allows kids to grow into the extra weight they're carrying, and it reduces the chances that they will get hung up on their bodies or on dieting.

Reduced need for insulin. Your child has type I diabetes. Once his "honeymoon" (the time after diagnosis when he is still producing some insulin) is over, all of his insulin needs must be met by injections. Since exercise lowers blood sugar, a child who exercises will require less insulin than if he wasn't active. Keeping insulin requirements as low as possible, consistent with good blood sugar control, is a good idea because it can mean a lowered risk of low blood sugars (at times when the child isn't exercising) and less likelihood of unwanted weight gain.

Emotional Benefits

Stress reduction. Kids need to blow off steam, let loose, get a little wild, and release the stresses of growing up. Exercise is a perfect answer to this need. You've probably had an experience like this: you're pulling your hair out because your child is bouncing off the walls. Suddenly you get a brainstorm: send him out to play. Half an hour later he comes back in, happy and relaxed. A miracle? In a way, maybe it is: a miracle you can create, which makes it extra special.

A better self-image. Kids need to feel good about themselves. A strong, healthy body that works as it should is one important source of those good feelings. Since your child has diabetes, he will almost certainly feel challenged in this area. That's why it's especially important that he be active; so he can enjoy the glorious, positive feelings that come when his body looks and performs its best. From the youngest toddler to the high school senior, these issues are front-and-center.

We know a pediatric endocrinologist named Dr. Raymonde Herskowitz-Dumont who works at the Joslin Diabetes Center in Boston, Massachusetts. Each summer she organizes Outward Bound adventures for young people with diabetes. She takes groups of kids 13 to 18 years old on sailing, canoeing, and scuba diving excursions. The kids are challenged physically, mentally, and emotionally. It is a very powerful experience for those who attend. They come away stronger and more confident not only in their diabetes management but also in every aspect of their lives. Not every child with diabetes can have the opportunity Dr. Herskowitz-Dumont offers, but participating in sports and active play can give them many of the same feelings that the Outward Bound kids experience.

Social Benefits

Bonding and identifying with friends. Kids want to have fun with their friends, and playing actively together is one of the best ways. It breaks down barriers and strengthens connections. It allows children to communicate without words. It teaches teamwork, sportsmanship, sharing, and healthy competition. It's just a wonderful way to relate.

Strengthening family ties. Chasing your toddler around the backyard, hiking through the woods with your 7-year-old, playing a game of pick-up basketball with your 11-year-old, or jogging a couple of miles with your teenager are all great ways to have fun and stay close. We'll talk a little later about how to make these family activities a regular part of your life.

THE RISKS OF EXERCISE FOR KIDS WITH DIABETES

While there are many exercise cautions for older people with diabetes, only a few of them really apply to children and teens. The risks of exercise for kids with diabetes include: low blood sugar, very high blood sugar, and foot injuries.

Low Blood Sugar

You're undoubtedly aware of the fact that exercise can lower your child's blood sugar too much, unless food and insulin are properly managed to prevent it.

It's important to keep in mind that your child's blood sugar can go low during play or exercise, immediately afterwards, or even many hours later. The lows during and immediately after exercise happen because the activity has burned up all the available glucose. Later, it may drop even lower. This delayed response is the result of the glucose reserves in his liver being used up while he was exercising. While he was active, his liver was breaking down stored sugar (glycogen) to free up glucose to fuel his play. For up to 24 hours after intense activity, his body will be trying to replace those fuel stores. Any sugar that gets stored in the liver or muscles is taken from the bloodstream, creating a risk for low blood sugar during the day following intense play or exercise. That's why it's especially important that your child eat all his scheduled meals and snacks in the hours after he's been active. He may also need extra food after he has played especially hard or long, even if he added snacks during the exercise.

Very High Blood Sugar

Not to make things too confusing, but another major risk of exercise is high blood sugar. If your kid exercises very strenuously, his blood sugar level may be driven up by the stress hormone adrenaline. Adrenaline is released during exercise to help make more sugar available to exercising muscles. A rise in blood sugar during exercise is more likely if your child's blood sugar is already high when he starts and he has very little insulin on board. When too little insulin is around, there is no way for sugar to get into the cells where it's needed to fuel activity. The cells, starved for fuel, signal the liver to make more glucose available. Sugar pours out of the liver but can't get into the cells because of the low insulin level. The blood sugar notches up even higher. Even though the blood sugar is so high, the cells still don't have any fuel, so they start burning fat for energy. This provides energy, but it also produces toxic acids called ketones. As ketones build up in the bloodstream with all that extra sugar, your child can develop ketosis. Not a good situation, to say the least. It's very similar to what happens when your child has a cold or the flu and his blood sugars get progressively more and more out of control.

Anytime your child's blood sugar is over about 250 mg/dl (check with your diabetes health-care provider to see what level he or she considers critical), he should check his urine for ketones. This is good practice whether he is planning to exercise or not, but it's especially important if he is about to be active. If he has no ketones, it's probably safe for him to play. With a blood sugar that high, however, it's still a good idea to take stock of where he is in the cycle of his insulin action. If his insulin is peaking or about to peak, he's probably fine; but if his insulin is running out, he needs to be more careful. Depending on the circumstances, he might choose to take a couple of extra units of Regular insulin, or he might just check again for ketones in an hour or so. If the ketone test is positive (especially if the quantity of ketones is anything above trace), he must clear the ketones with extra Regular insulin before being physically active. Follow your doctor's guidelines for supplemental insulin doses, but be very cautious about the dose if your child intends to keep exercising after the ketones are cleared.

Having ketones is rare for most kids. This is fortunate because testing for them is universally despised by people who have diabetes—adults and children alike. We're not sure why ketone test loathing is so deep and so common. Maybe it's the fact that it involves messing with urine or because it may signal a medical emergency. Who knows? What we do know is this: getting a child to test for ketones is sometimes easier said than done. If your child resists ketone testing, try some of the questioning and problem-solving techniques we discuss in Chapter 5. You might begin by conceding the obvious fact that your kid considers the whole process an unmitigated drag, and you might sympathize with him. Ask him how he would manage the situation. See if you can work out an approach together that doesn't seem overly burdensome to him. Your doctor or diabetes educator may have some additional suggestions.

Foot Injuries

Kids with diabetes have the same risk for all types of injuries that every physically active child faces, including the risk for blisters and foot injuries. Although diabetic kids have no greater risk for getting foot problems than their friends, their chances are a bit higher for having problems (like infections) with any injuries that do occur. This is because high blood sugars can interfere with normal healing, and they can slow down recovery from what would otherwise be only a minor irritation. This is another good reason to keep blood sugar as near normal as is safe and possible. Good footwear makes injuries much less likely and is a must for active kids.

MAKING ADJUSTMENTS

When your child is physically active, you and he will need to adjust his food intake, insulin doses, or both to keep his blood sugars where you want them. Blood testing is the key to making these changes safely and effectively. Insulin and food needs during exercise are affected by a lot of factors. To learn what works for your child in each unique situation, you must evaluate those factors: the time, length, and intensity of the exercise, your child's individual response to activity, the current blood sugar level, the insulin doses and timing, and the food that is onboard or planned. Armed with all this information, you can greatly reduce your child's risk of exercise-related high and low blood sugars.

When Is He Playing?

A Saturday morning baseball game, a prelunch dance class, an after-school bike ride, and an evening soccer practice will all require different approaches, because insulin availability and meals are different for each time period. You might deal with the risk of hypoglycemia during Saturday morning games by skipping or reducing your child's breakfast dose of Regular insulin or by adding more carbohydrate to his usual breakfast. The best approach for a prelunch gym class might be a larger midmorning snack, a little less morning Regular insulin, a little less morning NPH insulin (especially if the shot was more than 4 hours earlier), or some combination of these tactics. A lot of kids run fairly high blood sugars at the end of the school day. If this is your child's pattern, after-school activities may not take any special adjustments at all. On the other hand, this is the time that morning NPH insulin is working actively, so there are no guarantees. The later in the afternoon an activity takes place and the closer to normal the blood sugar usually is at that time, the more likely it is that less morning NPH and/or a bigger afternoon snack will be needed to prevent low blood sugar. Evening games often can be dealt with in the same way as morning games: reduced insulin (usually Regular) in the premeal shot and/or more food with the pregame meal. Insulin reductions, rather than food additions, are often preferred by very active youngsters, because they don't like to play on a full stomach. Naturally, learning exactly how to make these adjustments for your own child will take timely blood sugar testing and some trial-and-error practice runs.

How Hard Is He Playing?

Aerobic exercises, like soccer or swimming, cause a more dramatic drop in blood sugar than anaerobic activities, like lifting weights. Running track or cross-country will probably push blood sugars down more rapidly than less strenuous activities like archery. Experience will tell you just how big a drop in blood sugar your child experiences with each type of exercise.

How Long Is He Playing?

It's predictable that if your child plays an entire basketball game, his blood sugar will drop faster and farther than if he sits out most of the game on the bench. Of course, with team sports, chances are you don't know before a game exactly how much the coach will be using your child. When the actual amount of time played is very different from what you planned, it may call for an extra test or two and mid-game touch-ups of either food (more play than you thought) or insulin (much less play than you planned for). Although, to be honest, we don't know any kids who go along with taking touch-up insulin during a game!

What Is His Blood Sugar?

We've said it before, but we can't say it too often: timely blood testing is essential to avoiding low blood sugar in active kids. Active play without blood sugar testing is like flying blind: you might not crash, but your risk is really high. Ideally, your child should test every time he's about to play. If that's impossible (or he's unwilling), figure out with him the time closest to the starting whistle when he can test. If at all possible, he should have his meter handy, so he can check during the activity if he thinks he's low. Many kids, in fact probably most kids, resist testing during a game. If that's the case, they should be encouraged to eat something if they even suspect they are getting low. (See specific suggestions below and in Chapter 7). It's much better to risk being a little high than it is to let a serious low develop because of lack of treatment. Being high may mean he doesn't perform to his best ability. Being really low could mean the end of the game—at least for him.

What Is His Individual Response to Activity?

People differ a lot in terms of how exercise affects their blood sugar levels. You and your child need to pay attention to how he responds to exercise. We're not suggesting that he will respond exactly the same every time; there are too many variables involved for that to be true. But, if you keep track of patterns in your child's blood sugar levels when he exercises, you will learn a lot. The blood sugars will make more sense if you also record insulin doses and timing, the type of exercise, how long and hard your child played, his food intake, and anything else that seems to affect his blood sugars (illness, nervousness, arguments, or whatever). We know this is a lot of work, but it will really pay off.

How Much Less Insulin? How Much More Food?

After taking all those factors into account, decide whether you're going to change the food, the insulin, or both and by exactly how much. Generally speaking, reducing insulin also reduces the need for extra food during exercise, but it seldom eliminates it entirely. Remember, kids who don't have diabetes also eat and drink more when they're active. Here's some information and suggestions that should help you with the necessary decisions.

INSULIN AND EXERCISE

You may notice some specific exercise-related changes in how your child's insulin behaves. For one thing, the same dose of insulin may lower his blood sugar more while he's exercising than it does when he's less active. For example, a child whose blood sugar drops 50 points for each extra unit of Regular insulin when he's going about his usual school day (refer to information on the 1,500 Rule in Chapter 4) may find that each unit drops his sugar as much as 75 points when he's running cross-country. The only way to figure out the specifics for your child is to review blood sugar, exercise, and insulin records together.

Exercise also increases circulation, so his insulin may start to work more quickly than normal. The effect is strongest if he injects his insulin into a part of his body that he is vigorously exercising (his serving arm if he's playing tennis, for instance).

Guidelines for Insulin Adjustments

In people who don't have diabetes, the body reduces insulin during exercise to help make fuel more available to the muscles. We can't be as precise in reducing insulin as the body can be, but we can do a pretty good job. Both the timing and the amount of the reduction are very important. The following guidelines should help you work out the specifics of your child's insulin adjustments for different activities.

- For light activity of any duration or moderate exercise that lasts an hour or less, it is probably easier to make any needed adjustments by adding food rather than reducing insulin. (See **Guidelines for Food Adjustments** in this chapter.)
- For moderate exercise lasting more than an hour and for any very intense exercise, a combination of supplemental food and insulin reduction will usually provide better protection against low blood sugar than supplemental food alone.
- Reduce the right insulin. In general, you reduce the insulin that is acting most strongly (peaking) during the time of the exercise. This will vary with the exact regimen your child is on.
  - Morning Regular peaks between breakfast and lunch.
  - Morning NPH or Lente peaks between lunch and dinner.
  - Evening Regular peaks between dinner and bedtime.
  - Dinnertime NPH or Lente peaks between midnight and 3 A.M.
  - Bedtime NPH or Lente peaks around dawn.
  - Human Ultralente peaks about 12 hours after it's given.

- Regular insulin doses can be reduced a little, a lot, or even eliminated entirely, depending on how long and hard the exercise will be.
- NPH and Lente insulins are never completely eliminated. Start with a 10 to 20% reduction for exercise lasting over 60 minutes. Adjust up or down on the basis of blood sugar results.
- If exercise will continue all day (skiing, hiking, and other endurance activities), reduce the doses of all the insulins active during the day.
- Evening exercise can also be adjusted for by moving predinner NPH or Lente until bedtime. It may or may not be necessary to reduce the predinner Regular as well, depending on the exact time, intensity, and duration of the activity.
- Heavy exercise can reduce blood sugar for up to 24 hours after the activity is finished. If exercise is long or hard or takes place late in the day, you may also need to reduce the insulin that acts after the exercise is completed. For example, Todd played singles tennis all afternoon. To keep from going low while he was playing, he reduced his morning NPH by 30%. Then, to keep from bottoming out overnight, he also reduced his evening NPH by 20%.

The only way we know of to pin down the exact dose changes that will keep your child feeling and performing well is through blood testing: before, after, and often during exercise. We know the costs—both financial and personal—that go into blood testing. But we also know the benefits, because parents and kids tell us about them. And that's the main reason we're so sold on testing.

Guidelines for Food Adjustments

Even when insulin is adjusted downward for exercise, a small amount of supplemental food may still be needed. More substantial snacks are almost always needed when insulin is not decreased for exercise. Insulin may not be adjusted because the exercise wasn't planned in advance (a frequent occurrence with kids!), because the exercise is too short or light to call for it, or because your family hasn't gotten into making insulin adjustments yet. (If you aren't adjusting insulin yet, we hope you'll consider learning. It's a powerful tool for making life more normal and blood sugar control much more successful.) Here are some general guidelines for adjusting food, but just like insulin adjustments, the specifics will be unique for your child. You need to work them out through trial and error, based on blood sugar test results.

- About 15 grams of carbohydrate are needed to fuel each 30 minutes of moderate-level exercise in school-age children. The exact amount that is right for your child depends on body size (bigger bodies need more food for the same activity), the intensity of the exercise, and your child's individual response to activity.
- If blood sugar is below 100 mg/dl before exercise, eat a snack first.
- If blood sugar is 100 to 150 mg/dl, it's okay to exercise, but test again in 30 minutes (if the activity lasts longer than that) and eat a snack if blood sugar is below 100 mg/dl.
- If blood sugar is 150 to 250 mg/dl, it's probably safe to exercise without further blood sugar testing unless the activity is very intense or will last for longer than about 60 minutes, the insulin is peaking, or low blood sugar symptoms appear.
- If blood sugar levels are greater than 250 mg/dl, test for ketones before exercise. (See **Very High Blood Sugar** in this chapter for details.)
- If exercise is long or hard, extra food may be needed in the hours after exercise to prevent low blood sugar. The extra food is used by the body to replace storage forms of glucose that are used up during long, hard exercise.
- Fluid replacement is vital to both performance and to safety. Water is the best. Sport drinks (with 10% or less carbohydrate) are fine. So are fruit juices diluted half

and half with water. Sport drinks or juice will provide at least some of the carbohydrate your child needs to protect against low blood sugar.

RECOGNIZING AND PREVENTING LOWS DURING EXERCISE

Blood tests, together with food and insulin adjustments, will greatly reduce the number of exercise-related lows your child will have. Unfortunately, it won't eliminate them completely, so you need to be prepared. Treatment for low blood sugars that occur during exercise is really no different from treatment at other times, and guidelines for treatment are covered in Chapter 7. However, recognizing low blood sugars during exercise can be a bit tricky and deserves some special attention.

Some of the symptoms of hypoglycemia—sweating and increased pulse, for example—are also signs of an active workout. You and your child may overlook them, thinking that they're caused by the exercise. You'll need to work with your child to identify symptoms you both can rely on when he's hot and sweaty and short of breath from the exercise. You might start by listing all the symptoms that he ever has when he is low. Then put an "X" next to those that he also often has when he's active. Cross out the ones he rarely or never has when he is active. This can help him focus on his most reliable low blood sugar early warning signs.

It might also help to develop a checklist of circumstances under which low blood sugar is most likely: things like, "Blood sugar was headed down before exercise"; "Didn't test blood sugar before exercise"; "Insulin is peaking"; "Long time since last meal or snack"; and any others you and he have discovered to be important. Then you can remind each other to be especially observant when those conditions apply.

Help your child learn a simple (but difficult to follow) rule: If you feel hypoglycemic while exercising, stop. If he can, recommend that he test his blood. If he is low, have him eat or drink 10 to 15 grams of fast-acting carbohydrate—whatever he likes most and works best. You'll find more details on treating hypoglycemia in Chapter 7. Stopping, testing, and treating right away can be very difficult for a kid. But with your help, he can find the easiest ways to be safe. Go back to questioning and problem-solving if necessary. What foods or drinks is he most willing to carry and consume? What will help remind him to take his supplies with him when he heads out to play? Does he have any other ideas to make stopping, testing, and treating easier?

Here's a summary of our suggestions for preventing exercise-related lows:

- Test blood sugar levels before, during, and after exercise.
- If exercise is very intense or will last longer than an hour, decrease the insulin acting during, and in some cases after, the exercise (as described earlier).
- If possible, time activity so that intense exercise does not occur while insulin is peaking.
- Avoid using injection sites over muscle groups that will be heavily exercised.
- Have snacks handy during all physical activity.
- Eat or drink extra carbohydrate at least every 30 minutes during activity, if it is intense or lasts a long time. Sport drinks or fruit juices can fill this need while also providing needed fluids. Dilute fruit juice with an equal amount of water for better absorption of the carbohydrate.
- Take extra carbohydrate at the first sign of hypoglycemia. Test first, if possible. If not, take carbohydrate anyway.
- Eat more for up to 24 hours after exercise, depending on the intensity and duration of the activity and on blood sugar levels.
- Learn individual blood sugar responses to exercise.

EXERCISE FOR SPECIAL GROUPS OF KIDS

The Very Young Child

Active play is good for everyone, right down to the very youngest kids. There are, however, some special problems when it comes to incorporating exercise into the diabetes care plans of very young children. For one thing, little ones tend to play in short, spontaneous bursts. This makes methodical planning next to impossible. Instead of being able to prevent blood sugar swings by changing food or insulin before exercise, you're often stuck with coping with the lows that follow. In addition, very young children are less able to recognize that they're getting low and tell you about it. Because of this, parents and other adult caregivers need to be doubly watchful for signs of hypoglycemia when very little children are active.

For a preschool-age child, almost any activity can provide good exercise: walking around the block, riding a tricycle, splashing in the wading pool, romping at the park. Outings won't last long while your child is still very young. Even 20 minutes of active play at a stretch can give your child the exercise he needs...and increase his risk for low blood sugar. To make activity safe and enjoyable, you need to minimize that risk.

When your child is very young, avoiding and treating hypoglycemia is easier in some ways and harder in others. It's easier because your very young child is less likely to resent and resist your efforts to monitor and manage his blood sugars. He'll probably kick up less of a fuss than an older child might when you test his blood before he starts to play, stop him mid-play to give him a snack, or insist on a post-play blood sugar test. That's the upside. The downside is that your very young child probably can't recognize yet when he's getting too low. And even if he is able to tell when he's hypoglycemic, he may not be able to let you know that he has a problem. That's why it's especially important with little youngsters to install an early warning system.

Installing an early warning system. Your early warning system for low blood sugars has two parts: you and your child. Start right away learning to recognize subtle changes in your child's mood and behavior that signal dropping blood sugar. Then help your child learn to do the same as soon as he can. The signs you find to be most reliable may be unique to your child: an uncharacteristically grumpy mood, a sudden lack of coordination, a headache, feeling funny, or even unexpected sleepiness. As we discussed before, symptoms can be very helpful in avoiding problems, but they're never infallible. We hear all the time from parents who misread their child's behavior, assumed the kid was low (or not), and guessed wrong. Your child's feelings and behavior alert you to the possibility of low blood sugar. Testing is the only way to know for sure.

To add your child's watchfulness to the early warning system at the youngest age possible, guide him to notice how he feels when his blood sugar is too low. Each time you actually know he's low, ask him to tell you exactly how he feels. If he is unable to do this while he's low, talk about it as soon as he's feeling better. Keep it simple; he only needs one or two reliable symptoms to take care of himself. If he can't describe what he's feeling, try prompting him by asking if he's feeling shaky, headachy, sweaty, tired, or whatever other feeling you think might apply. It will take time before your child is able to recognize his lows, but it's never too early to begin helping him develop this essential skill. Once he gets the hang of recognizing that he might be low, he needs to learn to tell you how he's feeling. When both you and he are watching for the signs, your early warning system is in place.

Food and insulin adjustments for activity. Because activity usually comes in short, unpredictable bursts in very young kids, it is much more common to make adjustments for activity with food than with insulin. Because of their smaller body size and the fact that they don't engage in extremely strenuous activities, very young kids may require less carbohydrate to cover a given amount of active play than older youngsters. For example, our guideline earlier in this chapter suggests that most kids require 15 grams of carbohydrate for each 30 minutes of very active play. Preschoolers and toddlers often require much less, perhaps 5 to 10 grams for each 30 minutes of extra activity. Finding the exact amount your child needs can only be determined by using his records of blood sugar, food, and activity.

The More Serious Athlete: Organized Sports

Participating in organized sports can be a terrific experience for your child, helping him make new friends and feel good about himself. But it's not all a bed of roses. All of the concerns we've discussed, especially low blood sugars, are always on your mind. There are some tricks of the trade that may help your very active youngster.

Bring the coach up to speed. Your child's coach needs certain information so that your kid will have the best possible experience and you will have a bit more peace of mind. The bare essentials:

- Tell the coach what diabetes is.
- Explain that insulin injections, blood sugar testing, and extra food are necessary to its treatment and will be a factor at times during his play.
- Explain that your child can play safely and well, with certain precautions.
- Tell the coach how to handle any medical emergencies (small or large) that may occur.

If your child is young, his coach may have to help him with blood testing and treating lows at times. Some coaches are terrific: they deal with diabetes calmly and matter-of-factly and don't place any unnecessary limitations on the child. If your child's coach is such a person, you are blessed. If not, there's a lot you can do to help. First, you can educate the coach. Stick to the basic facts he or she needs to know. If you aren't quite sure what to say, check with your child's diabetes educator or other health-care provider. He or she probably has written material specifically designed to tell coaches, teachers, and others what they need to know. If information alone doesn't produce the desired result, try providing support as well. Be there to handle the extra tasks and to offer guidance and reassurance. Most people learn best from their own experience. If you help the coach be successful with your child and his diabetes, he or she will probably become much more confident and positive.

Depending on your child's age and level of maturity, he might want to talk to the coach himself or at least help with the process. It doesn't really matter who provides the information, as long as the coach gets what's needed. If at all possible, follow your child's wishes concerning his role. In most cases, it's wise to let your child tell his teammates. If he's not comfortable with telling the whole team, it's a good idea to make sure at least one buddy is in the know. This can be important to getting timely help with low blood sugar, in case the coach doesn't notice what's going on.

Get your child, his coach, and his teammates to see your child's diabetes in the same way: it's something he has to take into account when he plays, but it isn't a barrier to competition. With careful planning and good support, your kid can reach his athletic potential and goals with diabetes as surely as if he didn't have it. We know a teenager who has had diabetes since she was 2, and she is currently the second-ranked long jumper in the United States in her age-group.

Eating for competing. Food is fuel for competition. Fortunately, a healthy meal plan for a child who has diabetes—one high in carbohydrates and low in fat with adequate amounts of protein—is the same one recommended for most athletes. For an active young person with diabetes, healthy eating helps fuel exercise at the same time that it helps maintain good blood sugar control. A diet high in carbohydrates helps your child build and maintain adequate stores of glycogen in his muscles and in his liver. That's why eating well before, during, and after exercise is essential for your kid.

Table 8.1 summarizes how to manage food for competitive sports. As we've said many times before, everyone is different. Some of the suggestions listed in the table may

TABLE 8.1 Food Game Plan

Pregame Meal

- Eat the meal 1 to 3 hours before starting time.

- Aim for a meal high in carbohydrates with some protein and a minimum of fat. Protein and "Lente carbohydrates" (oats, beans, lentils, cornstarch) increase the protection against lows several hours after eating.

- Good food choices include lean meat, fish, or poultry, potatoes without gravy or pasta with tomato sauce, vegetables, bread (no butter), salad with fat-free dressing, fruit, and skim milk.

- Drink plenty of water or other fluids before the game, including 3 to 4 cups of fluid with the pregame meal and more to drink before the event. The importance of this is increased when outside temperatures are high and with greater intensity and duration of activity.

Snacks

- If the blood sugar is less than 150 before exercise, your child may need a snack of fresh fruit or fruit juice immediately before the game.

- For long and intense activity, your child may need a carbohydrate snack (approximately 15 grams of carbohydrate) during the game every 30 to 60 minutes. Sports drinks or diluted fruit juice may provide all or part of the needed carbohydrate.

- A postgame snack including carbohydrate may be helpful in warding off delayed exercise-induced hypoglycemia.

Adapted from Hornsby WG Jr (Ed.): *The Fitness Book for People With Diabetes.* Alexandria, VA, American Diabetes Association, 1994.

simply not be necessary for your kid, and others may not work well for him.

If your child wants to use a commercial sports drink, try one with less than 10% carbohydrate. If the carbohydrate in a drink is too concentrated (above about 12%, as is the case with regular sodas and undiluted fruit juice), the body can't absorb it as quickly. The result can be nausea, diarrhea, bloating, and discomfort. That's why we recommend diluted fruit juice (half water, half fruit juice) or a low-carbohydrate sports drink for carbohydrate replacement during exercise.

Carbohydrate replacement after exercise may also be a good idea for preventing hypoglycemia. Good choices are fresh fruit, low-fat crackers, muffins, granola, fig bars, oatmeal-raisin cookies, yogurt, soups, bread sticks, or pretzels. The extra food can be taken as an additional snack or added to planned meals or snacks.

Some kids are tempted to buy—or get their parents to buy—special meal supplements, power boosters, or vitamin and mineral formulas. Unless your child is missing some particular nutrient, these products are unlikely to provide any benefit—and they tend to be much more expensive than foods that provide the same nutrients. His strength, endurance, and athletic prowess will be the result of his natural gifts and the work he puts into his sport, not the result of any supplements he may consume. If he wants to learn how he can boost his performance, attending a camp devoted to his sport or consulting with a registered dietitian who works with young athletes might be a better investment.

If your child-athlete eats nutritiously most of the time, replaces carbohydrates on a timely basis, and takes certain precautions, he can learn through sports a tremendous amount about his diabetes, his body, and his life, which will stand him in good stead forever.

Kids who go overboard. Some kids, particularly in the preteen and teenage years, carry exercise too far. They become too competitive and push themselves too hard. These children go far beyond the requirements of good health in their commitment to exercise or athletic competition. All that's good about active play can become a problem when it is taken to an extreme. Overly competitive kids can feel worse rather than better about themselves, lose friends instead of making them, and hurt their bodies instead of strengthening them. This intense focus on exercise may arise from an extreme need to win, an overwhelming desire to be thin, or other factors.

Children who have diabetes certainly are not immune to these problems; in fact, they may be more susceptible to them than some of their peers, especially in the area of body weight concerns. They may be fighting the tendency to gain weight if their insulin doses are not well-regulated. Some youngsters use massive doses of exercise to fight this problem. This is a relatively rare occurrence, but it is a serious problem for anyone who has it. If you think your child is going overboard with exercise, try to talk to him to understand how he sees the situation. If these conversations don't allay your fears, you might want to talk to his coaches or to his diabetes health-care provider for further insight and advice.

Another way some adolescents who have diabetes try to control their weight is by taking less insulin than they need to cover the food they eat. This behavior, which we call insulin purging, is a form of eating disorder unique to people who take insulin. It's called purging because it's a way to purge or get rid of calories consumed, like vomiting or using laxatives. We talk more about insulin purging and other forms of eating disorders in Chapter 9.

The Inactive Child

Inactivity can be a temporary phase or a more persistent condition. Either way, it's a challenge to diabetes management and to overall health.

Some parents tell us their kids are classic couch potatoes. Their idea of exercise is using the remote control to channel surf or hiking out to the kitchen for another snack. If your child seems to prefer being passive to playing actively, there are certain things you can do to promote a healthier level of activity. But first, recognize that some kids will play less than others, no matter how much encouragement they receive. We don't think Einstein was spending his spare time mountain climbing. And chances are Bill Gates spent his childhood pennies on issues of *Scientific American* rather than new soccer balls. If your child is the contemplative sort, keep your expectations realistic. Enjoyable individual or casual pursuits (riding a bike, roller-blading, hiking through the woods) might have a better chance of captivating his interest than competitive or organized sports that require a major ongoing time commitment.

Work with your less active child to identify any form of activity he might enjoy. Time and money place certain limits on the available choices. But, with those constraints in mind, let your imagination and his take you where it will. Consider the possibilities. There's walking, dancing, biking (on the street or with a stationary bike at home or in a gym), aerobics, swimming, running, yard work, active housework, horseback riding, skating, skiing, rowing, all forms of team sports, bowling—the list goes on and on. Since it's obvious you can't exercise for your child, the activity he chooses has to be one he can live with. Use some of the problem-solving techniques we discuss in Chapter 5 to be an activity facilitator, to help your kid get going with exercise, and to help him maintain his motivation once he's under way.

You might offer to help in any way you can manage. Buying him some cool gear might do the trick, or taking him to games or lessons. But perhaps one of the most powerful tools you have is personally joining him in some of his activities. We know parents who walk, run, ride bikes, and play ball with their kids, and most often everyone seems to have a great time. Temper the choice of activity to the people involved. If Dad's a marathoner but Junior is an uncoordinated computer whiz who's barely seen the light of day all year, a grueling family power hike would probably be a big mistake.

Another problem we often hear about is the tremendous variability in activity level many kids experience over the course of the year. While the weather is good or while they are playing on a school team, some kids tend to be very active. In bad weather or off-season, the amount of time they spend playing drops abruptly. Sometimes, weekdays are active and weekends are not. For other kids, the reverse may be true. You know what a difference it makes in your child's control when he is active compared with those times when he's not.

The only way your child can avoid blood sugar control problems when he goes from an active phase to an inactive one is to make adjustments in other aspects of his regimen. For example, he can decrease the amount he eats or increase the amount of insulin he takes. Unfortunately, there are potential problems with either of these approaches. Eating less can be really difficult for some kids, especially those who already have problems sticking with a meal plan. If their level of activity is way down, however, chances are good that their appetite will decrease in response, at least to some extent.

Taking more insulin to make up for the reduction in activity is another option for keeping blood sugars closer to normal. Unfortunately, it can also lead to weight gain if your child is eating more food than his body really needs. Still, you need to make good blood sugar control a high priority. Work with your child to find an acceptable approach that has the most going for it and the least going against it. The best approach will probably involve both some reduction in food intake (see if your child's appetite points the way once the activity level is reduced) and some increase in insulin. It won't be perfect because it can't be perfect, but it will be the best you and your child can do. And you can continue to make adjustments and improvements any time the opportunity presents itself.

PERSISTENCE AND FLEXIBILITY

Unforeseen or unforeseeable situations are a fact of life with diabetes. Being physically active adds another level of complexity to the mix. But successfully meeting the challenges that active play and athletics present can build a degree of personal strength and diabetes know-how that is truly impressive. The answers won't be immediately evident. When we were young ourselves, kids used to have these little wind-up cars that would go until they hit a barrier like a wall or a piece of furniture. Then the car would bounce back and head off again in another direction. It looked as if the toy was trying to find a way around the barrier, constantly searching for a clear path. Those little wind-up cars are a great image for a kid with diabetes trying to reach his activity goals. Try one thing. If that doesn't work, try another and another until you turn enough corners to find the way.

HELP FOR EVERY ACTIVE KID WITH DIABETES

One wonderful source of information and motivation for any physically active person who has diabetes is *The Challenge*, the newsletter of the International Diabetic Athletes Association (IDAA). The IDAA has branches all over the world, and *The Challenge* describes the adventures and accomplishments of its members. The stories are interesting, informative, and inspiring. For more information about IDAA, write to

International Diabetic Athletes Association (IDAA)
1647-B West Bethany Home Road
Phoenix, AZ 85015-2507

or call

Tel: 602-433-2113
Fax: 602-433-9331

Beneficial as it can be to all children, exercise can be stressful at times for the child with diabetes and for those who care for and about him. Your child doesn't have to back off from exercise, or even from athletic competition, because he has diabetes. But he does have a lot more to think about and to plan and watch out for than his nondiabetic friends. And sometimes all his thinking and planning (and yours) doesn't do the trick, and he ends up with low blood sugar or some other diabetes-related crisis.

A friend of ours who's had diabetes for almost 20 years tells a story about an experience he had at college just after he was diagnosed. He was walking across campus after an intense racquetball match when he realized that he had no idea where he was. He was sure this made no sense, since he'd been in the same spot many times before. Then it struck him that he must be having his very first episode of low blood sugar.

He was desperate for something to eat or drink, but he didn't have any money. He approached a woman who sat on a nearby bench drinking a soda and tried to explain what was going on. Unfortunately, the sounds that came out of his mouth made no sense at all, not even to him. He grabbed the soda from the young woman and drained the can in a second. The woman leaped to her feet and went running across the quadrangle, screaming for help. Our friend quickly (and wisely) fled before anyone showed up to deal with the wild, soda-swilling terrorist.

He was actually able to laugh as he walked away, thinking about how ridiculous the whole scene had been. Add one more item to that list of supplies your child and you need to carry along when he goes out to exercise: food, testing supplies, medical I.D., and, oh yes, a sense of humor.

THE BOTTOM LINE

1. Exercise has physical, emotional, and social benefits important to all children.
2. The major risks of exercise for kids with diabetes are low blood sugars and high blood sugars. These problems can be prevented or minimized by a combination of blood testing and food and insulin management.
2. Food and insulin adjustments are unique to your child and the situation. They are based on the current blood sugar, when and what he ate, and when, how long, and how hard he will exercise.
4. Managing activity in small children is very challenging. Safety is enhanced by installing an early warning system for low blood sugars.
5. Diabetes does not need to be a barrier to competitive or strenuous athletics. Meeting the challenges of these activities is much easier if the coach and one or more teammates are aware of the needs of the child with diabetes.
6. Encouraging greater activity for the inactive child with diabetes is just as important as helping the athletic child compete successfully.

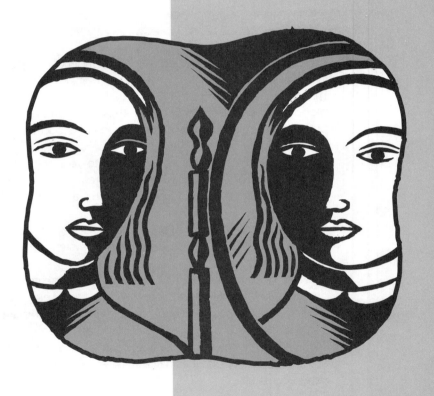

9 CHAPTER

· · · · · ·

"Jennifer is so thin, and she never eats with the family anymore..."

Recognizing Eating Disorders and Eating Problems

Jennifer finally admitted that she had been reducing her insulin doses because it helped her keep her weight down.

Jennifer was a senior, majoring in dance at the local high school for the performing arts. She'd been very active in her own care from the time her diabetes was diagnosed at the age of 8, and her blood sugar control had usually been quite good. All of that fell apart around the beginning of her junior year. From that point on, her control steadily worsened. By the middle of her senior year, her glycohemoglobin levels were almost twice normal, reflecting an average blood sugar of about 350 mg/dl. During the same period, her weight dropped from 135 pounds to 116 pounds. During the first 5 months of her senior year, Jennifer ended up in the emergency room three times because of ketoacidosis. Needless to say, everyone was very concerned about the problems she was having.

Jennifer's preoccupation with her weight had captured her dietitian's attention, and he decided to have a long, serious talk with the girl. After a lot of encouragement, Jennifer finally admitted that she had been reducing her insulin doses for months because it helped her keep her weight down. She was convinced that her success as a dancer depended on being thin. She said her problems dated back to her junior year, when she had begun cutting back on her insulin doses occasionally so she could eat less. She discovered that when she cut her insulin way back, her blood sugars shot up and the weight just melted away.

Twelve-year-old Aaron's parents were beside themselves with frustration. The boy just never acted satisfied with the amount of food they provided, and he seemed obsessed with eating sweets and other junk food. Every afternoon when he came home from school, he tried to convince his mother to give him a bigger snack. If he won, he greedily ate everything she gave him. If he didn't win, he'd sneak into the kitchen and get something more to eat anyway. Empty candy wrappers frequently showed up in his dresser drawers, under his pillow, or in his wastebasket. His teacher even called home once to report that he was trading parts of his lunch for candy and cookies. Although Aaron's weight wasn't a problem, his blood sugars were far from good, and he and his parents were bickering constantly about how to get his eating under control.

Jennifer had a serious form of clinical eating disorder unique to diabetes. Aaron's eating problem was less serious and far more common.

COMMON ISSUES AROUND EATING

Eating well is a challenge for many people, young and old alike, whether or not they have diabetes. Most of us, in fact, sometimes eat more than we should or eat things that aren't good for us. Why do we do these things even though we know they're not in our best interest? There are many reasons. For one thing, eating is pleasurable, and, for many of us, sweet and fatty foods deliver the most pleasure. Add to that the fact that eating is a social activity. Food is almost always included when people get together to have fun. We gather for breakfast, brunch, lunch, and dinner; for coffee and dessert; for pizza and beer; for holidays and birthdays; for weddings and funerals.

Skipping the food often means missing out on a lot more than just calories.

In addition, many of us are very attached to family traditions associated with food and eating. We want to eat the same dishes our parents and grandparents did. We want them to be prepared the same way they always were. Of course, old-time family-style cooking was not always the healthiest, but that doesn't change our desire for those foods. And as if all that wasn't enough of a challenge, every day, more and more people are turning to prepared foods and fast foods for family meals. Advertisers understand that. They know how little time is available for cooking anymore. They flood us with appealing messages to buy these easy, tasty foods. Unfortunately, many of those same convenient items are high in fat, sugar, and salt—not the best nutritional choices. Very few people eat right all the time. In fact, almost no one does.

Healthy eating can be doubly difficult for a young person, especially if she has diabetes. Your child wants to be just like her friends. She wants to be able to do what they do and to eat what they eat. But when she overeats or chooses unwisely, she suffers even greater consequences than her friends do. Just like them, she may have trouble controlling her weight when she strays off the nutritional straight and narrow. But she'll also have trouble controlling her blood sugars.

To be sure, not every child with diabetes struggles to the same extent with the issue of eating right. For some, the challenges are no different in type or degree than they are for those of us who don't have diabetes. They occasionally overeat, have difficulty staying away from junk food, and sometimes skip a meal or snack. But for others, the struggle is a truly desperate one, marked by bingeing and purging or severe restriction of caloric intake, disturbing and dangerous behaviors that indicate a clinical eating disorder.

CLINICAL EATING DISORDERS

Clinical eating disorders are the most serious but least common. If your child spends a lot of time thinking about what she should eat and managing her eating, that's probably just a sign of good diabetes self-management. And a concern with eating and weight are common in our society, especially among young women. But these facts mean that kids with diabetes are almost certainly quite focused on what they eat. In addition, many people who have diabetes, especially the young ones, feel that simply by virtue of having a chronic disease, there is something wrong with their bodies. Put these forces together and you get a strong tendency for young women between the ages of 14 and 30 with diabetes to be preoccupied with what they eat, how they look, and how much they weigh. A smaller number of young men in the same age range have similar problems. Unfortunately, in some of these young people this preoccupation leads to a full-blown eating disorder.

The problem of eating disorders in people with diabetes has received quite a bit of attention in the past few years. There is some evidence that eating disorders may be more common in young people with diabetes than they are in the rest of the population. Whether this is true or not, we know that there are some unique features to eating disorders in diabetes. We also know that when they do occur in diabetes, the consequences are very serious indeed.

Eating disorders come in two forms. One, anorexia nervosa, involves a severe self-imposed restriction in caloric intake, often combined with extreme levels of exercise. The other, bulimia nervosa, involves binge eating followed by purging, usually in the form of vomiting or the use of diuretic medications or laxatives to get rid of the extra calories taken in during the binge. Diabetes offers another possible form of purging. By reducing or omitting insulin after binges, the child with bulimia and diabetes can drive up the blood sugar, causing calories to wash rapidly out of the body in the urine.

Obviously, having either type of eating disorder enormously complicates diabetes management. In fact, there's really no way a person who has anorexia or bulimia can take good care of her diabetes. People with eating disorders are almost always in terrible metabolic control, and they often spend lots of time in the hospital. Those who have bulimia usually have chronically high blood sugars, and they may end up in the emergency room with ketoacidosis due to omitting insulin. Those with clinical or subclinical anorexia, on the other hand, usually have low blood sugar levels most of the time, and they may even need to be hospitalized for recurrent and severe bouts of hypoglycemia. There is evidence that people with eating disorders tend to have problems with virtually all parts of the diabetes regimen: blood sugar testing, taking insulin on schedule, following a meal plan, maintaining adequate blood sugar control, fitting exercise into their treatment regimen, and so on.

We know one young woman who became convinced of the value of tight control shortly after her diabetes was diagnosed. Unfortunately, she carried a good thing too far. She dramatically reduced her eating, restricting herself to 1,100 calories a day. She tested her blood often, and her average reading over this period was around 60 mg/dl. She went for almost 2 years with glycohemoglobin levels below the lower limit of normal. She also was having a lot of low blood sugars. More than once, she required emergency medical attention to bring her back from a more severe episode. Her approach to diabetes care certainly was dangerous, but she was so preoccupied by fears of gaining weight and developing complications that she found it impossible to ease up on her regimen.

Clearly, both anorexia and bulimia carry major risks for short-term problems with diabetes control. Furthermore, studies show that young people who have eating disorders and a history of poor metabolic control develop complications (particularly retinopathy and neuropathy) earlier and more frequently than people who don't have an eating disorder. In addition, some researchers have found that even people with less serious forms of eating disorders have worse metabolic control and more complications than those who are clearly free of these problems. This means that any disordered eating behavior is cause for concern and should be treated seriously.

How to Recognize an Eating Disorder

How can you tell if your child has an eating disorder? The first step is to understand what's normal. Then you have a point of reference for judging behaviors that are troubling and need to be evaluated by a professional. To begin with, it's very understandable that many children in our current society are interested in their weight. This isn't exactly what we would classify as normal, although it's certainly common. Young boys and girls should be playing, not chatting with their friends about cellulite. But our children are exposed to many "thin is in" messages—especially via advertising and the mass media—from a very young age. The value put on thinness is so prevalent that it's almost inescapable. This is not dangerous in itself, but it can cause great stress and self-doubt for those who don't fit the Madison Avenue mold of what's attractive. As we've said before, this desire is much more common among young women than it is among young men. This is probably related to the much stronger link our society makes between a woman's appearance and her worth than it does between a man's appearance and his worth. As much as we might deplore this and worry about young women growing up in this climate, it's not something that we're likely to change or solve easily.

Given this environment, however, we can say that it's understandable to want to be slender. Further, it's normal for a person who wants to be thin to be disappointed if she is not. It's also normal to exercise to manage weight and stay fit. It's normal to overeat occasionally (or even fairly often). And it's normal to eat prunes or use other approaches to manage occasional constipation.

It isn't normal—and may indicate that your child has an eating disorder—if

- She weighs less than 85% of the normal range for her height, body frame, and age.
- She has an intense fear of gaining weight or being fat, even though she is already underweight.
- She sees herself as fat when others say she is too thin.
- She exercises far more than is necessary to stay fit.
- She misses at least three consecutive menstrual cycles (in young women).
- She denies the seriousness of her low body weight.

- She binges (eats very large amounts of food at a single sitting) at least twice a week for 3 months.
- She feels she can't stop eating or control what or how much she is eating.
- She induces vomiting.
- She uses laxatives, diuretics, or enemas to lose weight.

In the realm of diabetes, it's normal to adjust insulin doses to maintain good blood sugar control. It is not normal, and strongly suggests your child has an eating disorder, if she purposely takes less insulin than she needs to maintain good blood sugar control with the conscious intent of managing her weight. Insulin manipulation is an especially troublesome form of eating-disordered behavior, unique to people with diabetes. It is frighteningly frequent. In fact, some researchers estimate that as many as 50% of all young women with diabetes frequently take less insulin than they need in an effort to control their weight.

Severely restricting eating, bingeing, purging, and manipulation of insulin doses can have disastrous consequences, leading to acute emergencies and contributing to chronic complications. For many young people, however, the appeal of thinness is so great that it makes all the risks involved in an eating disorder seem acceptable.

Young men also suffer from eating disorders. However, the far more intense pressure toward thinness that is placed on young women in our society is confirmed by the fact that eating disorders are about 10 times more common among women than they are among men.

Kids almost never acknowledge this type of problem voluntarily; in fact, they usually go to great lengths to cover up what's going on. People who have an eating disorder hide what they are doing because they're terrified that someone might try to force them to give it up. And they're often deeply ashamed.

The tendency of those with eating disorders to cover up their behavior is not the only thing that can make it hard to know for sure whether they have a serious problem. It can also be challenging to distinguish between a normal (and even positive) focus on food and fitness and the abnormal concerns and behavior that reflect an eating disorder.

Pay close attention to your child's behavior to see whether you find any of the signs of a clinical eating disorder. If you do see such signs, first talk to your child to see if she is willing to confirm that there is a problem. If she acknowledges that she's struggling, that's a good sign. Take action right away to get her the professional help she needs. We make this recommendation even though we know it's difficult for you to be sure whether your child has an eating disorder. And we know it's even scary to admit that she might have one. In spite of these feelings, it's important to get help for your child if you even suspect she might be suffering from an eating disorder. Even milder forms of disordered eating can lead to serious problems with diabetes management. Talk to her diabetes health-care provider and ask for a referral to a mental health professional who treats eating disorders and, hopefully, also knows something about diabetes. This kind of professional should be able to evaluate your child's situation, using screening questionnaires and a clinical interview, and treat your child if she does have an eating disorder.

Some Types of Treatment

If you live in an area where there is a large diabetes treatment center, your child may be able to participate in a diabetes clinic-based group treatment program for eating disorders. The successful programs of this type are generally conducted jointly by the medical and mental health staff associated with the clinic.

Trained mental health professionals can also choose from a variety of individual psychotherapies, which have been shown to be effective for some. You need to understand, however, that for many reasons, overall success rates are not high. One form of psychotherapy, called cognitive-behavioral therapy (CBT), addresses the thoughts, feelings, and behaviors associated with emotional problems, including eating disorders. Young people undertaking CBT to deal with an eating disorder work to modify their extreme beliefs about weight and body shape. This process is called cognitive restructuring. Recently, some researchers have reported successful treatment of eating disorders using the new class of antidepressant medications known as selective serotonin re-uptake inhibitors (SSRIs). One of the drugs in this group is Prozac.

Regardless of the type of treatment chosen, hospitalization is often necessary. Medical hospitalization is required if the young person is malnourished or suffers from a mineral imbalance. These problems are more common with anorexia than with bulimia. Psychiatric hospitalization may be required to normalize eating behavior and to treat any associated psychiatric problems, such as depression, especially if the young person is suicidal.

If Your Child Denies the Problem

If your child doesn't acknowledge that she has a problem, but you're still worried, talk to her diabetes care provider for further advice. In addition, be sure your child knows the following things:

- You love her very much.
- You are concerned that she might have an eating disorder, and there are reasons for your concern.
- You are available to talk about the issue any time she wants to.
- You are going to talk to her health-care provider about your concern. You can suggest that she might want to do the same, if she is ever worried herself. You might also encourage her to talk to any other adult she trusts: a relative, teacher, religious advisor, or coach.

Ways to Prevent Eating Disorders

Given how devastating an eating disorder can be, you're probably interested in anything you can do to prevent your child from developing one. While there are no guarantees, there are some things you can do (or not do) that can help. How much they will help depends a lot on your particular situation. Remember, most kids aren't vulnerable to eating disorders. For those who are, their parents' approach to their eating, weight, and diabetes care can make a difference. First, be sure that you take a flexible, individualized approach to your child's diabetes management—the kind of approach we describe throughout this book. If this is a real issue in your family, it may be helpful to re-read Chapters 1, 2, and 5. If you insist on rigid or perfectionistic standards of food and blood sugar control, a susceptible child may respond by binge eating or avoiding food. Moreover, if you push too hard for tight blood sugar control, your kid may gain weight. Then, if she finds that disturbing, she may begin skipping insulin in order to get her weight back down.

You may also need to examine your own attitudes toward weight. If you make a big deal about it for yourself or for your child, that can add to the pressure she feels to be thin. Remember, Madison Avenue hype aside, everyone is not programmed genetically to have a model's lean and lanky look. There are many people who are stocky or heavy, even when eating and exercising reasonably. Being comfortable and accepting helps your child to truly like her body and to feel comfortable with the shape nature provided. A susceptible child may still have problems because of the prevailing culture or the remarks and biases of her peers, but body criticism can be particularly stinging when it comes from parents. In addition, think about the example you provide. Do you have a relaxed and healthy attitude toward your own eating? A positive value for fitness rather than a tense preoccupation with the scale? Do you binge or diet restrictively? Parents who do have such issues risk transferring them to their kids. They need to get help themselves in order to help their children.

LESS SERIOUS EATING PROBLEMS

As we've said, almost everyone has problems with eating at one time or another. Now we're talking about garden-variety problems, not those sure-enough psychological disorders like anorexia or bulimia. By garden-variety problems, we mean very common and not too serious issues like occasionally eating too much, difficulty in resisting favorite unhealthy snacks, or struggling to stick to a regular schedule of meals and snacks. Temptation, habits, social pressures, and stress all contribute to these problems. Obviously, your child feels the same kinds of pressures. And when she does, she may stray from the healthy eating plan or practices you and she worked out with her diabetes health-care provider. Different kids will stray to different degrees and in different ways. For some children, sticking with the meal plan is relatively easy. They don't seem to be that tempted by things that aren't on the plan. They're happy eating what's better for them, and they're not particularly drawn to the sweet and high-fat foods that can interfere with healthy eating. They work out ways to manage social situations like parties and sleep-overs without feeling awkward or deprived. Unfortunately, these kids are in the minority.

The majority of kids with diabetes get hung up on some aspect of their nutrition at least occasionally. They overeat, gobble up things they shouldn't, or refuse to stick to a schedule. As we pointed out earlier, these types of problems aren't unique to people with diabetes. They are human and common. That's not to discount the amount of hassle they can lead to when conscientious parents get upset by the way these behaviors can sabotage blood sugar control. The key to dealing with and minimizing these problems is to follow the parent and child job descriptions, which we first talked about in Chapter 1. They will help you avoid making mealtimes a battleground. You want your child to grow up feeling that eating is relaxed and unpressured, not a source of criticism, deprivation, and stress. You need to work with your child to make mealtimes good times. For example, in your effort to get the right food on the table, try to accommodate her tastes to a reasonable degree. We're not suggesting you cater to her every whim, cooking special meals on a regular basis. This can make you into a short-order cook and, if you're not careful, can make your child demanding and manipulative. But we are suggesting that you include some of her preferred foods in the choices at every meal and not force her to eat anything she absolutely loathes. Avoid going to war over cleaning up a plate.

Remember also that once you get the right stuff on the table, it's the child's job to decide exactly what and how much to eat. Children won't always choose exactly what you'd prefer, but as we discussed earlier, you can usually deal with this by offering choices instead of ultimatums. And what about the child who wants to eat the same thing all the time? Don't worry about it. We know a kid who ate spaghetti with meat sauce, string beans, and applesauce every night for 27 days in a row. Nothing terrible happened, and peace reigned. The same principle applies to breakfasts and lunches. Your child can eat the same cereal every day for weeks or the same type of sandwich for days. It's the whole selection of foods eaten from day to day that determines good nutrition, not the 14th peanut butter sandwich lunch in a row. Look at the forest, not the individual trees. Use the Diabetes Food Pyramid to make sure the necessary groups are being included. If the overall intake is reasonable, the boring sameness of limited preferences can actually contribute to better blood sugar control by eliminating food as a variable. You can bet that by the third or fourth time that kid had eaten spaghetti, green beans, and applesauce for dinner, his parents had a lock on the right insulin dose and timing!

We know that having some of your child's favorites available at every meal may mean extra work. Only you know how much of this is really possible in your situation. Some things may be easy to make along with any other food you are preparing. Others may be prepared in quantity and stored in the refrigerator or freezer for use over time. If she loves chicken, you could broil or bake enough at one time to provide her four or five dinners. You might also be willing to make her a healthy sandwich in place of part of a meal she doesn't like. As your child gets older, she will be able to do an increasing amount of meal preparation for herself. This can begin very simply: she can get the box of cereal from the shelf (assuming she can reach it) and bring the bottle of milk to the table when it's okay for her to substitute cereal for part of her meal. When she's older, she can boil the water to make her own pasta, prepare her own sandwich, or heat her own vegetables.

For many parents, the hardest part of applying this approach is getting past the feeling that the child should eat whatever is put in front of her. For some, it's almost a moral issue. For others, it's just an extension of the way their parents handled food. While expecting a child to like every food that's offered sounds admirable as an abstract principle, in practice, it is often a disaster, whether a child has diabetes or not. And when a child does have diabetes, things are potentially even worse. A kid with diabetes is already dealing with more than her fair share of eating issues. What she really needs is less pressure and the opportunity to make choices. She's much more likely to make healthy eating choices now and later if she feels she has some control over the situation. Restricting her choices only makes it more likely that she will rebel and eat out of control.

Think of your own goals, as well. You want your child to be healthy and happy and to learn how to take care of herself, unencumbered by major food hang-ups. You also want mealtimes to be peaceful family occasions, not food fights. You are much more likely to accomplish your goals if you let your child make as many choices as possible, choose from the foods that you provide, and eat what her appetite dictates. Keeping insulin and food in balance while taking this approach is a challenge, but the benefits to family relationships are significant. While you are the only one who can decide exactly what's possible for you, we encourage you to stretch a little in this regard. We think you'll like the results.

Some Tricks to Smooth the Road

Plan meals ahead of time. Planning ahead can make following the parent and child job descriptions much easier. Some planning will be done well before mealtime. For example, try talking with your child before you do your weekly shopping to get her input on the menu and the shopping list. This can help ensure that at least some things she wants will be on the table. Make this a regular part of your routine so you both know the drill. If your child doesn't seem thrilled by the prospect, don't push it. Wait for the time when she's looking for something that's not there and suggest that she (or you) put it on the shopping list. Or, if she's willing, take her with you to the grocery store. Be clear beforehand that you will have veto power over any purchases she might suggest, but that you will try to be flexible. Some parents swear by having an occasional special shopping trip with their child just to buy the things she needs for snacking, treating low blood sugars, and so on. This isn't something you need to do every week, of course. It's just a way to ease your child into the meal planning process.

Finally, planning also takes place on the day of the meal. To avoid last-minute glitches, check with your child to be sure that you're including things in the meal she wants to eat. That way, if she's unhappy with the menu, there's still time for one or both of you to make adjustments. Does all this sound like a lot of work? We won't deny that it is, but it's a lot less work and a lot more productive than making mealtimes into a battleground.

Eat what you want your children to eat. Your food-related attitudes and behavior affect your child's eating habits. If you tend to overeat, delight in junk food, and continuously nibble, it's unlikely that your kid will have much luck controlling her own eating. We know that puts extra pressure on you, and since you (probably) don't have diabetes, you might think that this is unfair; that it's all right for you to eat as you do. Unfortunately, it's not that simple. It's hard to help a child develop good eating habits, even under the best of circumstances. The task becomes nigh to impossible if your message is, "Do as I say, not as I do."

What should you do if your own eating patterns are not the best? We can think of a couple of possible choices. You may be able to think of others. One option is to keep eating as you do and acknowledge openly to your child that you are not living up to the standards you want her to meet. This may come back to haunt you when you try to get her to do the right thing, but at least this approach has the advantage of honesty. The other option—and the one that we have found to work best for most families—is to accept the challenge to change your own behavior. Change is difficult, but your efforts could bring great rewards: better health for you and for your child and a closer relationship.

If you do choose to change your own eating behavior, do it sensibly and gradually. Going on a crash diet won't work, and it sends your child the wrong message, as well. Follow the healthy eating guidelines in Chapter 3. You might also want to consult a nutritionist if you are having problems getting started or if you feel you need extra help and support for any reason at all.

Control the environment. Environmental control can be a big support in maintaining healthy eating habits. Most people we know find they are more likely to stick to their meal plans if they put on their plate only the amount of food they are planning to eat, and then leave the rest on the stove. We think this is a great idea, as long as you stay flexible and are able to provide more food if appetites warrant it. Also make sure that the amount you're portioning out is appropriate—remember, if a child is either hungry all the time or leaving a lot of food uneaten, the meal plan probably needs adjusting. Eating family-style, with a whole plateful of meat, a loaf of bread, a bowl of vegetables, and everything else on the table, can be a set-up for overeating. You and the kids may keep eating to "clean it up," not because you're really still hungry. While the approach of sitting down with only the food you intend to eat may be easy for some families to manage, it will be awkward or difficult for others. Still, it can help you keep track of exactly how much is eaten, and it keeps the business of portion control off the table. Consider giving it a try. Another environmental technique is keeping junk food out of the house or buying it in small quantities that are likely to be eaten at a single sitting. If it ain't there, it's hard to eat it!

Don't expect perfection. You'll also help to minimize your child's eating problems if you check out your expectations for her behavior (refer to Chapter 5 for additional suggestions). Perfection is no more a possibility when it comes to your kid's eating than it is in blood sugar control. Parents who expect perfection often find that their children become overwhelmed by the unrealistic standard and then just say, "To hell with it. I'm blowing it anyway; how much doesn't matter." But, of course, how much does matter. Or they may begin to hide what they're really doing from parents who they know would be upset by the truth. The challenge is to be both ambitious and realistic. Try to make your goal very good eating and very good blood sugar control. But be flexible. There are lots of choices to be made as your child learns to take good care of her diabetes. Help her see that she still has a lot of good choices, even though her diabetes limits them somewhat. Ask her questions about the food-related situations she finds hardest to manage, and then really listen to the answers. Ask her what makes these situations easier to take or when they are less difficult than usual. Find out if there's anything you can do to help. Help her learn to control her own blood sugar. A flexible, accepting, problem-solving approach will make that far more likely than fruitlessly demanding perfect behavior.

Follow your job description. Get help if you notice signs of disturbed eating. Most important of all, love her as she is, support her in becoming all she can be, and make sure you two stay on the same side of the fence. Keep clear about your role: You cannot do more and you should not do less.

THE BOTTOM LINE

1. Most people sometimes eat more than they should or eat things that aren't good for them. The severity of such problems ranges from garden-variety issues about food to full-blown clinical eating disorders.
2. Young people with diabetes, especially young women, are at higher risk for such problems.
3. Young people who have diabetes and a clinical eating disorder (anorexia nervosa or bulimia nervosa) are almost always in terrible blood sugar control.
4. The symptoms of a serious eating problem include low body weight, fear of being fat, excessive exercise, abuse of laxatives, binge eating, and self-induced vomiting. If you notice any of these symptoms, it's vital to get help.
5. A mental health professional who treats eating disorders can evaluate the situation and provide treatment, if needed.
6. Parents can help prevent both garden-variety and more serious eating problems in susceptible children. This requires successfully managing their own eating and attitudes about food and weight and following the parent and child job descriptions described in Chapter 1.

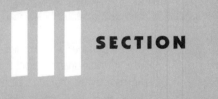

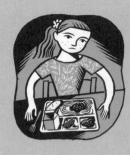

The third section of the book describes how to apply what we know about feeding and nutrition to good diabetes care at each stage of development.

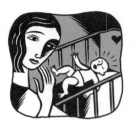

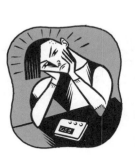

Food, Diabetes, and Development

The third section of the book describes how to apply what we know about feeding and nutrition to good diabetes care at each stage of development. Chapter 10 deals with babies and toddlers. Hypoglycemia is a major concern in these very young children. Special issues for infants include how to manage fluids and starting solids. As babies grow into toddlers, avoiding fights over food becomes important. We describe how to support your toddler as he begins to feed himself and how to deal with the ever-present "No!" Chapter 11 focuses on preschool and school-age children. Challenges multiply as children spend more time away from Mom and Dad's watchful eye. Ideas for informing others—school personnel, parents of friends, etc.—about your child's diabetes are included. We discuss testing and managing hypoglycemia and injections at school, dealing with school lunches, parties, fast foods, and sleep-overs. Chapter 12 deals with the challenging teen years. Adolescence is a particularly rocky time for parents and youngsters to work together on diabetes management. Driving, drinking, drugs, and sex are touchy subjects for every family, but their implications are even greater for the teen with diabetes. Techniques for staying involved enough to ensure your child's safety while still promoting growing independence are included.

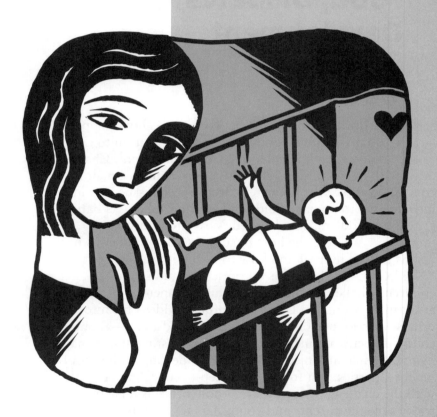

"It seemed like I'd just finished feeding, diapering, and testing his blood, and there he was, crying for the next feeding."

Babies and Toddlers

What if a cry
meant he was
hypoglycemic
instead of just
wet or hungry?

Corey was only a little over 2 months old when his diabetes was discovered. As is often the case when children develop diabetes before they're old enough to tell people how they're feeling, he had gotten really sick before anyone realized something was seriously wrong. He had to be admitted to the hospital because of DKA (diabetic ketoacidosis: a very serious condition caused by lack of insulin). He was "limp as an old dishrag," according to his mother. The pediatrician and nurse were very sympathetic and willing to help, but since babies with diabetes were pretty rare in their small, agricultural town, the professionals didn't have much practical advice to offer about Corey's day-to-day care.

"You'll just have to do a lot of blood tests," the doctor informed them. "That's the only way we can figure this out. Test before and after every feeding, before you put him down to sleep, and anytime he's acting unusual."

Since Corey was their first child, the young parents didn't have a real handle on exactly what the doctor meant by "unusual" behavior, so there was a lot of testing going on, at least at first. What if a cry meant he was hypoglycemic instead of just wet or hungry? But the number of tests dropped off very quickly once they realized the costs involved. They just couldn't afford to do the number of tests the doctor recommended. Their HMO provided one vial of test strips per month. That didn't even get them through the first week after they brought Corey home from the hospital. Once the free vial was gone, every additional test was a tough decision, because at 70 cents each, the costs added up very quickly.

The young parents didn't have a real handle on exactly what the doctor meant by "unusual" behavior.

• • • •

Besides the cost of the tests, the young couple had trouble dealing with the disruption they caused. Corey's mom hated doing a blood test before feeding him because the baby got so upset. He'd always been an eager feeder and didn't tolerate a lot of dallying around once he decided he was hungry. The delay in his feeding and the further indignity of being stuck in the heel added up to a totally unacceptable situation in the babe's view. As his dad described it, he "went nuclear." Mom and baby were both a wreck by the time she sat down to nurse. She was afraid the upheaval was interfering with her milk supply and so was skipping as many of the blood tests as she felt she could. Since Corey was being breast-fed, he was nursing every 2 to 3 hours on average. With feedings so close together and so many things to do with each one, no one was getting much rest. Blood sugar control was poor, which was generating 12 to 15 wet diapers a day. More disposable diapers, more expense, more stress. And the baby wasn't gaining any weight. No one knew for sure whether this was due to the disruption of Corey's feeding, to a real problem with Mom's milk supply, or to the diabetes itself (because of poor blood sugar control).

After close to 6 weeks of this roller coaster, Corey's pediatrician was feeling just about as overwhelmed as his thunderstruck parents. It took several heated phone conversations for the doctor to convince the HMO that the family needed to be seen right away by a pediatric endocrinologist in the nearest large town.

Corey's story highlights several issues that are very common for families with diabetic babies. First and foremost, Corey's mom and dad were feeling terribly uncertain and overwhelmed: the almost universal reaction of parents whose infants develop diabetes. Caring for the baby was taking up nearly all of their waking hours. They worried about hypoglycemia constantly and wondered about the meaning of every cry, burp, and twitch that the baby emitted. They were uncertain about his food intake and were challenged both emotionally and financially by the other demands of Corey's care. Also, the medical personnel in their town didn't have much experience with diabetes in babies.

This can be a problem, even in fairly large cities, because there aren't that many babies with diabetes. Most children develop diabetes at a later age. Even doctors who see a fair number of older children with diabetes may have very little hands-on experience with a small infant. This can be a problem because certain aspects of care are unique to this age-group. If the team caring for the diabetes doesn't know the tricks of the trade, parents need to learn them the hard way, by trial and error. But, because infancy is fairly brief, the child may grow into a whole new set of issues and challenges before the parents have really mastered the ins and outs of their baby's diabetes management.

Every family with a diabetic infant also faces the challenge of balancing the need to know the blood sugar level against the cost and discomfort of testing. Understandably, everyone we know absolutely hates to stick a baby. For most families, the younger the child, the more angst surrounds both shots and blood tests. Turn up the stress meter a few more clicks. And yet the test results provide extremely important information, because the baby can't tell you if he's feeling sick, low, etc.

Finally, the questions and concerns that surrounded Corey's feedings are also typical for families dealing with diabetes in an infant. The milk feeding—whether it's breast milk or formula—is the sole source of nutrition for babies younger than 5 or 6 months of age. How it's managed is absolutely vital to the baby's overall health. But the details of how to keep the milk and the insulin in balance are neither easy nor obvious.

This all sounds pretty daunting, and it is. But there are some tips and techniques that can lighten the load.

BABIES

First of all, rest assured that your baby with diabetes is going to grow and develop normally. Keeping blood sugars in reasonable control helps ensure this. Your doctor will track your baby's growth on a grid, similar to the ones shown in Figures 10.1 and 10.2. Growth grids are explained in Chapter 2. But here's a caution about them that's especially pertinent in infants: lengths (heights) are often taken incorrectly. Babies squirm. They resist being stretched out on those little measuring tables. Lengths recorded for squirmy babies are often inaccurate. And even when babies get big enough to stand, things might not get much better. If the pattern on the growth grid doesn't make sense to you, take it with a grain of salt or ask the doctor or nurse to measure again. If your baby is gaining steadily, has strength and energy, is nursing and eating contentedly, and doesn't seem particularly hungry or lethargic, that's pretty powerful evidence that he's doing fine.

There may be a short setback in development right after your baby's diabetes is discovered. This is true of babies who have any kind of health problem. Once this little blip is past,

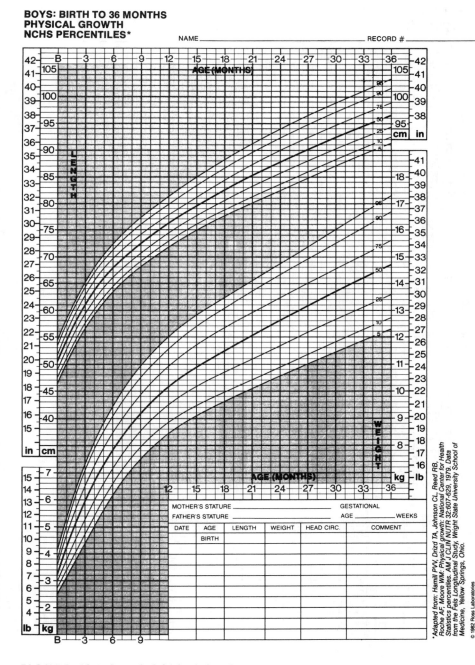

FIGURE 10.1 Growth Grid for Infant Boys.

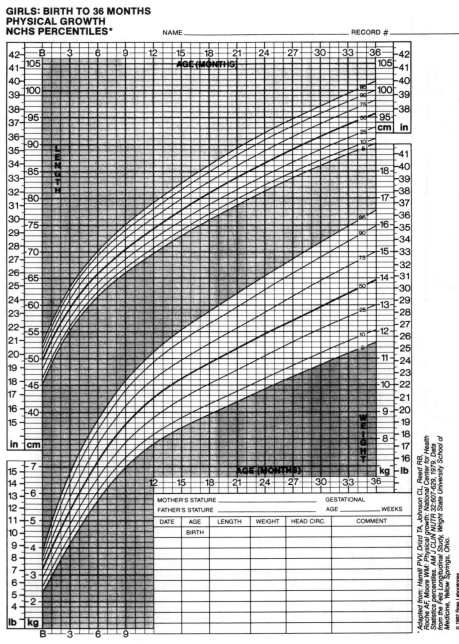

FIGURE 10.2 Growth Grid for Infant Girls.

all of the developmental milestones of infancy—sitting up, walking, talking, and so on—should happen according to your baby's proper timetable.

Your baby with diabetes needs lots of love, care, closeness, and nurturing—just like every other baby. Some of the closeness will now be connected with diabetes care routines—in particular, shots and blood tests. Parents tell us there are tricks that help take some of the sting out of these tasks. Making the daily pokes with needles and lancets less stressful can do a lot to help everyone's frame of mind. And from a nutritional viewpoint, keeping everyone a bit calmer promotes smoother feeding.

Here are some words of advice from parents who've been there. Avoid sneak attacks to do shots and finger or heel pokes. Babies and older kids alike may get paranoid and start to flinch every time you pick them up for a cuddle. Instead, consider setting up a diabetes care station where you keep the supplies. Do all the shots and blood tests there while you're at home, at least until your child gets older and more accepting of the routine. Distract the baby at the critical moment or have someone else do it: patting or squeezing another part of the body works well; so does offering a favorite toy. Use plastic pipettes to transfer blood from heel or finger to the strip. This cuts down both on having to control a squirming baby and on wasting strips because of an ill-timed kick or lunge. When you're done, cuddle immediately and thoroughly. If the child has gotten teary or upset, cuddle until he's calm before trying to nurse or feed him, if at all possible. And purchase a meter that requires a small blood sample, not a big, hanging drop. There is a newer meter that allows an accurate reading when a small sample is rubbed across the test strip. It includes a visual confirmation that enough blood was used (Sure Step, Lifescan, Inc., Milpitas, CA).

Blood tests are the only way to confirm low blood sugar, and regular blood tests are vital to knowing your baby's pattern of control. But extra blood tests sometimes can be avoided by doing urine glucose tests, cutting costs and tears. This is an option when your main concern is high blood sugar. Urine glucose testing doesn't give you a specific blood glucose number, but it does allow you to confirm high blood sugar. For example, if your baby is wetting more diapers than usual, leading you to think he's running high, you can often confirm that the sugar is high with a urine test. You may be able to do a urine catch at the time of a diaper change. If not, you can wring a few drops of urine out of a wet cloth diaper or diaper liner (most disposable diapers that "don't leak" contain silica gel, which makes it impossible to squeeze urine out of them). Not perfect, but a helpful bit of information gathered at a smaller cost—both financial and personal. Don't forget, however, that there can be a time lag between actual blood sugar and a urine test result. If the urine you're testing was made some time before you do the urine test, the blood sugar may have had time to drop in the meantime. That time lag and other uncertainties are why we never adjust insulin on the basis of urine sugar. Urine either from the diaper liner or from a urine catch done at changing time can be used to do urine ketone tests as well. Your doctor will tell you when these are needed—most likely anytime the baby is sick or has very high blood sugar.

Hypoglycemia in Infants

Low blood sugars are scary and potentially dangerous in infants. That's why most doctors and parents set somewhat higher blood glucose goals for infants and very young children than are common for school-age and older kids. Keeping blood sugar a bit higher—say, making 100 the lowest acceptable blood sugar—gives you a margin of error that will cut down on the number of lows. This is one of the most effective ways of protecting your baby against excess low blood sugars.

Another important prevention tactic in babies is to not force-feed. When parents force, it almost always leads to babies actually eating less. This is true both of the milk feeding (breast-feeding or formula) and of solids, once they're started. Be alert to your baby's signs of hunger—for example, the type of cry that distinguishes hunger from a wet diaper or from general fussiness. Then offer breast, bottle, or solids in a calm, matter-of-fact fashion. Hungry babies will usually eat. If the baby takes much less than usual (appetite does vary), be on the alert for signs of dropping blood sugar. Most babies nurse or eat willingly when their glucose level is dropping.

Insulin management in babies is tricky. They don't eat major meals the way we do, and their intake is variable and all but impossible to change. For these and other reasons, most doctors don't use any Regular insulin in babies and toddlers. Two or three injections of intermediate- or long-acting insulin spread your baby's insulin out as evenly as possible through the day. This is well-suited to the way babies graze, eating and drinking small amounts several times throughout the day. Because not using Regular insulin means fewer strong insulin peaks, it provides some protection against low blood sugars. Blood test results help you and the doctor keep the baby's insulin doses adjusted to his food intake and to the changing needs created by growth and development. Insulin adjustments in babies need to be very small—often half-unit changes are made. Even half a unit is a lot of insulin in a tiny little body. Bigger dose adjustments may lead to radical changes in blood sugar. It's not uncommon to dilute insulin to make it possible to give very small doses accurately. Your health-care provider can teach you how to do the dilution and how to measure doses correctly for the specific dilution and syringe you're using.

Even with careful insulin management, hassle-free eating, and modified blood sugar goals, babies will still become hypoglycemic at times. And, of course, they can't tell you what's going on. It helps to become familiar with your baby's particular symptoms of falling blood sugar. There are a lot of possibilities. Your baby might have a particular cry, become pale or cranky, start to sweat or tremble, or develop a bluish tinge to fingers or lips. Symptoms are your early warning system. They are your sign to test. If you can't test, treat anyway. It's safer than waiting to see what develops. Brain development requires a constant supply of glucose. Preventing low blood sugars in infants, whose brains are still developing, is a very high priority. It's also vital to treat low blood sugars as quickly and effectively as possible. This ensures that the blood sugar doesn't stay low for any longer than is absolutely unavoidable.

To treat low blood sugar, offer a drink with easily absorbed sugar. Apple juice seems to be a common standby, but anything that works well for your baby is fine. It probably won't take a lot. Carbohydrate goes much farther in a small body than it does in a larger one. One Fruit Exchange or a 15-gram portion of carbohydrate is often used to treat hypoglycemia in school-age children and smaller adults. Is it any wonder, then, that a mere 5 grams (the amount in about 1 ounce of juice or 2 ounces of sugar-sweetened Kool-Aid) usually does the trick for a little baby? Once the blood sugar is back up, follow the sweet drink with formula or breast milk to keep the blood sugar up. In older babies who are taking solids, cereal or bread with some egg or other protein could be offered as a follow-up instead of a milk feeding.

Glucagon is needed if the baby won't eat or if the treatment doesn't seem to be working. Glucagon is discussed in detail in Chapter 7. Every home with a baby who has diabetes needs to have glucagon (this advice is true for every age-group!).

Feeding Infants

The milk feeding. From birth until about 4 to 6 months of age, the milk feeding is the baby's only source of nutrition. Either breast-feeding or bottle-feeding with formula will produce a healthy baby. If you're breast-feeding when your baby develops diabetes, balance what you and he are getting out of breast-feeding against the reassurance that some parents and doctors seem to get out of being able to actually see how much the baby has taken from a bottle at any given time. If you're trying to make this decision right now because your baby has just been diagnosed with diabetes, keep this in mind: trying to wean a baby from breast to bottle when you're also dealing with your feelings and the unfamiliar demands of diabetes care won't make the adjustment any easier. If you do decide to go on breast-feeding, be aware of Mom's stress level, rest, fluid intake, and nutrition. Problems in any of these areas can interfere with the milk supply. In some cities, if the baby is admitted to the hospital at diagnosis, this decision may be taken out of your hands and the baby placed on formula to simplify things for the hospital staff.

Starting solids. A baby needs solid foods for the first time at around 4 to 6 months of age because his nutritional needs are changing and because his development demands it. He's getting to the point where he can coordinate tongue and jaws in such a way that swallowing solids becomes possible. The strong gag reflex of infancy is receding. He becomes able to sit up without support. The stage is set to move on to his next phase, eating semisolid and solid foods. Giving solids at younger ages doesn't have any nutritional benefits.

When solids are first started, practicing the skill of eating is actually more important than the foods themselves. The milk feeding should still be the major source of nutrition. Solids shouldn't really displace the milk feeding until a child is well-established on a variety of table foods. This generally happens somewhere around 1 year of age, or a bit older.

Because the first nutritional need to be met by solids is that for iron, the preferred first solid food is fortified baby cereal. It should be given by spoon in a semisolid consistency. Each 2-tablespoon serving prepared with milk provides about 5 grams of carbohydrate. At about 6 to 8 months, fruits, fruit juices, vegetables, and "finger breads" (teething biscuits, arrowroot cookies, etc.) can be added one at a time. Two-tablespoon servings of fruit provide about 4 to 5 grams of carbohydrate, as does each ounce of fruit juice. There is no real need to include protein foods this early, since the baby will still be getting adequate protein from the milk feeding. Meats and eggs can be added at around 7 to 10 months, when the baby begins to graduate to table foods. Sometimes, it's very tricky to figure out how much a baby (or toddler) has actually eaten. Do you count what's smeared on the high chair? No, but how do you know how much got past the lips versus how much ended up as wallpaper? We don't have an answer. Parents of the youngest children with diabetes seem to favor retrieving food from faces, trays, and bowls and reoffering it for as long as the baby is still eating willingly. An inexact science at best. But we can tell you that smearing, spitting, and throwing generally escalate after the child's had about enough. Take stock of how much was eaten before the pablum hit the fan.

There is no reason to give babies artificially sweetened drinks. They get plenty of sweetness from fruits and fruit juices. Some families of diabetic infants use sugar-sweetened Kool-Aid or punch to treat low blood sugar, which is fine. But using artificially sweetened drinks when the baby is just thirsty may unnecessarily encourage a preference for sweets. Plain old water is probably the best additional beverage for babies, beyond the milk feeding and the small amount of fruit juice needed to meet vitamin C needs and to treat an occasional low blood sugar.

As the baby's meals become more substantial, moving carbohydrate around in the day can help keep insulin demand in balance with insulin availability. For example, if high blood sugars are a problem at mid-morning, some fruit, fruit juice, or starch could be moved from breakfast or the morning snack to noon or later, when the morning NPH, Lente, or Ultralente shot will be having a stronger effect. Vegetables or meat could be given in their place in the morning feeding. These choices would still satisfy the baby's hunger but have less effect on blood sugar.

TODDLERS

A mother that one of us works with has observed that dealing with her toddler was nature's way of preparing her for teenagers—a wise woman. There are, indeed, some similarities between the two. Toddlers are proving to themselves and to you that they are separate people. Teenagers are trying to prove the same thing to the whole world. Resisting you is an excellent way to prove that separateness, and so a toddler's favorite word is no! He very much wants to explore and be independent, but at times, it scares him to death. Your job at this stage is to let him explore, help him be successful as he tries new things, and yet set clear limits. Without limits, the 2-year-old and the teen will push and push until you're forced to step in. Setting and maintaining reasonable limits is also important in feeding the toddler.

Toddlers Do Best With Lots of Choices

This is the age of self-feeding, so make food easy for him to eat on his own. Give him his food already cut into bite-size pieces. Leave the dressing off his salad so he can eat it with his fingers. Stay away from things that are too dry or tough for him to manage easily on his own. Remember the parent and child job descriptions from Chapter 1? You get the right stuff in front of the child and decide when, where, and how (mealtime behavior) the meal or snack will take place. The child decides how much he will eat of what you offer. Reminding you of this with regard to the toddler is very important, because trying to force a toddler to eat is like poking a short stick into a pile of sleeping rattlesnakes. You will not be happy with the result! Avoid fighting and scolding during meals at all costs. This will have a negative

---

Trying to force a toddler to eat is like poking a short stick into a pile of sleeping rattlesnakes.

● ● ● ●

---

effect on your child's intake in both the short and the long term. The best way we know to keep the peace is to have plenty of acceptable choices available: choices that you know your toddler enjoys and that meet the current demands of diabetes control. When your main concern is getting enough food into the child to cover insulin, offer some different choices or bigger portions of things you know your child enjoys. On the other hand, when the toddler has eaten all the planned meal and is yelling for more, offer choices with less blood sugar impact, like proteins, fats, and low-carbohydrate vegetables.

This is the age when children learn how to manage silverware. Keep in mind that all learning starts with not knowing, so they'll be total klutzes at first. Show your child how it's done by doing it yourself. Praise him for whatever he's able to manage reasonably well. He'll pick it up eventually by watching you and practicing, so be patient. Putting too much pressure on having great table manners at this age may distract the child from eating.

If your limits on what, how, or how much is eaten are too rigid, there may be tremendous battles (food fight!), and your child's nutrition, as well as his attitudes about food, could suffer. But the same will be true if you don't set limits. Maybe your limits at this age include 1) coming to the table with the rest of the family, 2) sitting in the chair while eating, 3) choosing what he wants from what's offered, and 4) not whining, hitting, or throwing food. If such basic rules are violated, it's fine to ask your toddler to get down. Refer back to Chapter 5 for ideas on how to handle the diabetes realities of this. Some parents tell their youngsters, "I warned you already that you can't scream during dinner, so you'll have to get down. But you may drink your milk before you leave if you like." Faced with expulsion from the family circle and being offered a choice (not told "Drink that milk before you leave the table because I'm worried sick about you having low blood sugar!") apparently works fairly well in getting a bit of protective carbohydrate into the child before he leaves the table.

Appetites and Schedules Change in Toddlers

Appetite is likely to be reduced during the toddler stage because growth is slowing down. Your toddler is probably putting on some height, but not much weight. Part of his energy needs are being met from burning his baby fat. Portion sizes for toddlers are shown in Chapter 3. They're small. For example, just 16 ounces of milk and an ounce of meat give a toddler all the protein he needs in a day. With these tiny needs in mind, give a little less than you think he will eat. If he asks for more, it's his idea, and he's more likely to eat it than if you put it on the plate and then try to urge him to clean it up!

Babies are fed pretty much on their own schedule. In the toddler stage, on the other hand, your child will be joining the rest of the family in a regular schedule of meals and snacks. Having adequate time between meals and snacks is one important way you can help make sure that your child is actually hungry when he sits down to eat. Uncontrolled snacking between meals can reduce appetite at mealtime, leading the child to refuse to eat. That makes arguments more likely and will probably compromise his overall nutrition, since snacks may not include all the Pyramid food groups to the same extent that regular meals do.

Don't Push Sweets, Milk, or Juice

With all children, it's important to avoid making sweets and other foods into rewards. This is doubly important for the child with diabetes. Food is given even greater emotional power when it is used as a reward. Whether you're rewarding a child for some accomplishment or for good behavior, try to use nonfood items (stickers, small toys, hand stamps, hugs, kisses, praise). These things don't affect the blood sugar, complicating your management tasks further. But perhaps more importantly, they help avoid creating a strong connection in your child's mind between food and being rewarded. This will keep paying off throughout his life, with reference to both diabetes control and weight management.

Also, don't push juice and milk on your toddler. These foods are important, but they shouldn't be given in quantities that compromise your child's appetite for the other foods he needs. Like the infant, the toddler will do best to use water to quench thirst. Artificially sweetened drinks are certainly safe, but some people feel that giving them instead of water just reinforces a sweet tooth.

Insulin and Blood Glucose Monitoring in Toddlers

Insulin management in toddlers is very similar to insulin management in infants. Regular insulin is used quite rarely. Strong insulin peaks are avoided as much as possible. If your child is eating in ways that create significant blood glucose peaks, try moving the carbohydrate foods around (offer fewer choices or smaller portions when you're trying to minimize carbohydrate) to bring down the peaks. Most doctors prefer to delay adding Regular insulin to the regimen until a child is well into grade school. If you can keep postmeal blood sugars in reasonable control by spreading carbohydrate throughout the day, so much the better.

To make shot times more peaceful, give the toddler some tasks and choices to help with the process. A toddler can choose where to get the shot or wipe off the spot with a swab. As described earlier, insulin can be given after the meal if your toddler's appetite or intake are quite unpredictable. This is not a perfect solution, of course, but will probably produce at least as good blood sugar control as guessing at the dose before the child eats. Its big advantages are that it reduces parents' worries and cuts way down on mealtime battles fought to make a child eat enough to cover his insulin.

Blood glucose monitoring is very important. Toddlers are still generally unable to recognize and warn you about developing lows. Test results are also vital to keeping your toddler's insulin properly adjusted to his food intake. Some of the stress around testing can now be defused because the child is getting old enough to participate more actively in the process, if he chooses. Toddlers can choose a finger to stick, pick out a lancet, or pick out a test strip from the vial.

Low blood sugars often become more of a challenge in toddlers because of their increased activity. They're so excited by this new skill of getting around on two feet that they seem to run everywhere. This is a big change from infancy. Insisting on regular meals and snacks, keeping juice or whatever readily available for treatment, and having an eye like a hawk are all helpful in cutting your toddler's risk for low blood sugar.

THE BOTTOM LINE

1. In infants and toddlers, goals generally are set to avoid high and low blood sugar rather than to achieve a near-normal level of control.

2. Hypoglycemia is the biggest fear of parents. Recognizing and preventing it are the biggest management challenges in very young children.

3. Symptoms of hypoglycemia can include crying, pallor, sweating, being cranky, and trembling. Symptoms are your sign to test the blood sugar.

4. A small amount of a sweet liquid, such as apple juice or sugar-sweetened Kool-Aid, given by bottle or cup, is the best treatment option.

5. Either breast-feeding or bottle-feeding can provide adequate nutrition for an infant, and both are workable with diabetes control.

6. Solids are started at about 4 to 6 months of age, when babies are developmentally ready. High-carbohydrate foods (cereal, fruit, and fruit juice, for example) can be moved around in the day to help correct patterns of high or low blood sugars.

7. Toddlers are self-feeders and are trying hard to prove they're separate people. Avoid hassles by letting them choose from appropriate options and by offering foods in a form that helps them feed themselves.

8. Toddlers begin to move into the same meal schedule as the rest of the family.

9. Growth slows in toddlers, so energy needs and appetite drop. Portion sizes are small.

10. Don't push sweets, milk, or juice. Kids don't need large amounts. Too much can destroy their appetite for other foods.

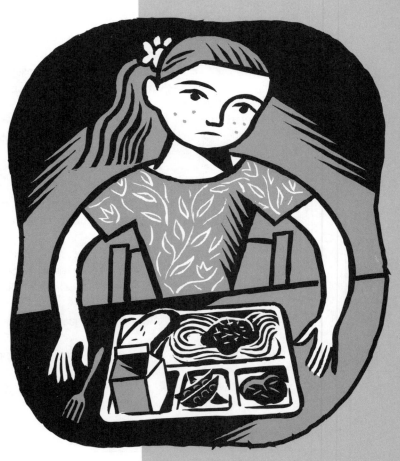

"Now she eats away from home at least as much
as she eats with us..."

Preschoolers and School-Age Children

It wasn't the first time that Kate had been the victim of a school lunch program that didn't always produce what the menu promised.

Eleven-year-old Kate's auburn hair was the first thing most people noticed about her. So thick it needed special barrettes to catch it up in her preferred ponytail. It bounced grandly as she marched into the dietitian's office. "Guess what," she said with a twinkle in her hazel eyes. "I must have had six Starches for lunch today. I bet my blood sugar's 300!" It wasn't the first time that Kate had been the victim of a school lunch program that didn't always produce what the menu promised. "I know I shouldn't have eaten it all, but I was real hungry, and they didn't have any more meat or salad."

This problem came up occasionally, even though Kate and her mother dutifully reviewed the school's menus at the beginning of every month. They marked the calendar with which days would be school lunch days and which would require a lunch from home. Some of the decisions were based on what Kate liked (chicken

223

fingers) and disliked (beans and wieners). Others were based on their experience with particular meals, like the cafeteria's spaghetti, which always sent Kate's blood sugar straight to the moon.

The biggest problems happened when the cafeteria ran out of the main dish and substituted something entirely different. The substitutions weren't always great for diabetes control. Once, the cafeteria workers had offered beans and wieners in place of the promised hamburger. It might have worked, except for the fact that Kate hates beans and wieners. She didn't eat enough to cover her insulin. Predictably, she had low blood sugar during the last period of the afternoon that day.

On the day of her visit to the dietitian, the low-carbohydrate chicken fingers meal had been replaced by spaghetti with marinara sauce and a roll. Kate was quite right. She had at least six Starch Exchanges, and her blood sugar was over 300 mg/dl when we tested it in the office. Her mother had spoken to the cafeteria staff about these last-minute substitutions several times, but the problem still seemed to surface occasionally. Sometimes the staff just forgot to set a meal aside for Kate before they ran out. Other times, substitute workers weren't aware of her needs. Short of sending all of Kate's meals from home, they hadn't found a foolproof way to solve the problem.

As children grow into the preschool and school-age years, they often take their first real steps out of the ever-watchful gaze of Mom and Dad. More and more of their meals and activities take place away from home. Mom isn't able to control the portions or the type of food that her son is offered at friends' houses. Dad isn't there during physical education class to notice his daughter getting pale as she runs the full length of the soccer field for the tenth time. Field trips, overnight stays at friends' homes, all-day jaunts to the mall or an amusement park; your growing child is facing choices and temptations that weren't part of the picture when more of her life was lived nearer to home. The complications for diabetes management multiply with each new experience. Parents are constantly trying to balance the child's need to grow and become independent against her equally important need to be safe. The process may have started even earlier, as in babies and toddlers who attend day care. But certainly by the age of about 4 or 5, most children are spending some time (and eating at least some meals) away from Mom and Dad. The frequency and the variety of these new experiences grow all through the elementary school years.

Many challenges are likely to surface for the first time between the ages of about 4 and 12. Television's influence on kids' food preferences and activity level increases tremendously. The family must deal with the need to share diabetes information with a wider and wider circle of people. The child must be kept safe at school and in other settings, without being overprotected or singled out for special treatment or unwanted attention. Reliable and acceptable ways to manage insulin and blood testing away from home must be found. Parties and sleep-overs need to be managed so that diabetes doesn't interfere unduly with the child's enjoyment of normal activities. And while dealing with all these changes and challenges, it's important to promote the child's progress toward greater independence in self-care. Uncertainty is the name of the game. Every change may mean a new schedule to adjust to, a new skill to acquire, or a shift in responsibility between parent and child.

When you have an infant with diabetes, all her care is totally in your hands. As a toddler, a child is able to participate in small ways in some aspects of care—making food choices from what's offered, picking the lancet for a blood test, or choosing where to give an insulin shot, for example. Then come the preschool and school-age years, where the child develops the mental capacity and maturity to begin the long process of learning to control her own blood sugar. Your task is to help her make the transition, sharing responsibility in ways appropriate to her development, style, and circumstances. This allows her to keep growing in independence and skill. And—of equal importance—it ensures that you stay involved so that her safety is protected while she learns the skills and develops the maturity to take over completely some time in the future.

SHARING INFORMATION ABOUT YOUR CHILD'S DIABETES WITH OTHERS

Because preschool and school-age children range farther and farther from home, it becomes necessary to share information about diabetes with more people. Children vary tremendously in their openness and comfort in sharing that information with adults and other children. Your child's own personality and acceptance of diabetes and your family's general communication style all play a role. So does her relationship with the people being told, their style and response, and the amount of time spent with them. How much, when, and who will be told are decisions that must be made by each family. There will be some people who must know, in order to ensure your child's safety: the teacher, coach, bus driver, and the adults in any house where she will be spending a significant amount of time, for example. There may be others whom you or your child just want to inform. Use the questioning and problem-solving techniques described in Chapter 5 to help your family identify the best decisions for you.

PRESCHOOLERS

The preschooler is a breath of badly needed fresh air to parents who have survived the antics of the testy toddler. The 2-year-old struggled against everything to prove her separateness. The 3- and 4-year-old defines that separateness as a happy little moon orbiting around Mom and Dad, who have become the center of the universe again. Preschoolers are generally positive, energetic, and eager to please. They are figuring out what it means to be human, and their main way of doing that is to imitate Mom, Dad, and older siblings. Their drive to imitate means that parents' food choices have a particularly strong influence on the child's own food preferences during this phase. Just like you'll eventually hear whatever you say come out of a 3-year-old's mouth, you'll eventually see whatever you eat be put into it!

A preschooler's limited attention span and great need to be active and explore go hand in hand with her limited ability to sit still for very long. Therefore, long, formal meals will be a trial for everyone. Instead, expect a preschooler to eat with gusto and focus for just about as long as she's actually hungry. Once the edge is off the appetite, she's likely to begin to dawdle or want to head off on other pursuits. Her imagination is developing rapidly, and she may have difficulty distinguishing between real and make-believe. Logical, critical thinking comes later, so she probably can't consistently make the connection between her actions and their consequences. That's one of the reasons why meals and snacks need to be planned and made to happen by Mom and Dad. In the preschool stage, a child simply doesn't think ahead to the probable consequences of skipping a snack or playing harder than usual. Mom and Dad are still the brains of the operation at this point.

The preschooler's eagerness to please can help along your efforts to shape her food preferences.

● ● ● ●

The preschooler's eagerness to please can help along your efforts to shape her food preferences, so take advantage of it. Get the right foods into the house and onto the table. Set the meal times and rules for behavior. For the most part, the preschooler will go along with the program. If she strays, refuses, or makes mistakes, just say no. Be polite but firm. Don't make it personal, and avoid shame and guilt. Because your approval and good opinion are so important to her, she's likely to go along with you most of the time, provided these things do not become a battleground. Notice it and congratulate her when she tries to do the right thing. If you criticize her efforts, she may stop trying because she doesn't want to disappoint or anger you. If she's afraid to make mistakes (in food choices or table manners, for example), she'll have trouble learning what she needs to. Mistakes are part of the learning process.

Eating Style

The shape, texture, size, and color of the food offered to the preschooler are very important. She will accept moist foods more readily than things that are dry or tough because they're easier to chew and swallow. Cut her food into manageable pieces, but be aware of shapes, because she may be. Anyone who has ever cut a peanut butter sandwich into little squares for a 3-year-old who was expecting little triangles has learned this important lesson! Because of their stage of mental development, most preschoolers don't really grasp that the same food cut up into different shapes is still the same food. They focus on what they see, and little squares are different from little triangles. Logic will get you nowhere. Logical thinking doesn't come along for a few more years.

Table manners and food-handling skills improve slowly but surely through the preschool years, but they still don't reach real mastery. A 5-year-old can probably get through dinner without spilling the milk but may still have trouble managing knife and fork, depending on the food. When setting expectations for mealtime behavior, take your child's level of coordination into account. Expecting more than the child is capable of will increase everybody's stress level, and it still won't make the 5-year-old as coordinated as an 8-year-old.

Structured Meals and Snacks

Having diabetes in the family tends to keep everyone tuned in to the importance of regularly scheduled meals and snacks, and this meets the preschooler's needs beautifully. If you plan and schedule defined meals and snacks, you help your child develop a more predictable pattern of hunger and satisfaction. When this happens, she will eat more consistently and willingly, a big boon to diabetes control. To help ensure that she has an appetite for meals when they're offered, limit snacks to the regularly scheduled ones as much as possible. Make sure that there's enough time between meals and snacks to allow her to get hungry for each one. Avoid offering juice, milk, or other caloric beverages between meals and snacks. They tend to curb the appetite.

What if your child begs for more food right after a meal? If she ate her meal and is still hungry, providing more food is probably the right thing to do. To help with blood sugar control, offer things that are less likely to raise blood sugar: nuts, peanut butter on celery, beef jerky sticks, low-fat cheese, or other low-carbohydrate items. On the other hand, if the child refused the previous meal (even though some choices were available and the consequences of not eating were explained), it's best to take a harder line. Kids need to learn to live with the fallout of their actions, whether it is being hungry until the next scheduled snack or having low blood sugar. Letting this kind of situation play out at home is a safe and responsible way to help your child learn the importance of eating her regularly scheduled meals and snacks. It's much more effective than yelling and trying to force the child to eat to prevent an undesirable outcome. And, in most cases, it's also much less stressful for all involved. When the consequence comes, the teachable moment is at hand. The preschool years are not too early to start this, and it is an approach that retains its effectiveness from that point on.

Another option for a child who picked at her meal and later comes panhandling for a snack is to offer her leftovers from the previous meal. This prevents kids thinking they can fish around for something better if they refuse a meal.

Insulin and Blood Glucose Monitoring in Preschoolers

There's nothing unique about insulin and blood glucose monitoring in the preschooler. Insulin regimens tend to remain much like the toddler's. Sensitivity to Regular insulin remains high, and if it is used at all, the proportion of Regular in the regimen tends to be quite low. Blood glucose monitoring continues to be very important, because food intake may be low or erratic at times and because the child is still too young to reliably recognize developing low blood sugar and inform you about it.

SCHOOL-AGE CHILDREN

There's a reason why formal schooling starts at around age 6 or 7. This marks the child's development into the realm of rational, concrete thought. Tremendous learning took place earlier, to be sure: walking, speaking, social skills, coordination, and so on. With that background taken care of and a reasonable command of language, the school-age child is ready to learn about the wider world. Her curiosity is tremendous. Her social interests become directed outside the family. She is able to follow rational lines of thought and appreciate cause and effect. As a result, she can begin to be responsible for her own actions.

She becomes physically able to perform virtually all the diabetes self-care tasks by about age 10, but she is still developing in terms of her emotions and maturity. This makes it important that parents stay involved in daily care, to make sure diabetes management doesn't fall by the wayside when the child does the expected: when she behaves like a child! During the school years, her ability to recognize and inform you about developing hypoglycemia should become well-tuned, and she probably will be able to select and administer her own treatment for mild low blood sugar episodes. She is able to understand the effects of various foods on her blood sugar and can make appropriate food choices, even when Mom hasn't laid out all the right foods in all the right portions. Not that she will make the best choices all the time. The lure of being just like her friends or of eating foods she never gets at home is sometimes just too powerful. But she can now understand the probable outcome of her choices, and she can learn from the experience.

As at all ages, really, desired behaviors can best be encouraged in the school-age child by catching her doing something right and praising her for it. It's also very valuable to recognize her efforts, even when the outcome isn't everything you might want. Try out new ways to deal with all the challenges that come with the developmental spurt in the school-age years. Whether these experiments turn out well or turn out poorly, they're the best way to learn. Keep talking with your school-age child about her diabetes management. Ask her what's working and what's not, what she wants, and what bothers her about her diabetes. Stay involved in the process and try to convey a positive, supportive outlook. This helps your child do the same. It will also pay big dividends when your child becomes a teenager.

Catch her doing something right, and praise her for it.

● ● ● ●

Anything that has been a source of stress or hard feelings in the school-age child is likely to explode into a full-blown battle during the teen years. If you have been able to establish a comfortable, cooperative approach to diabetes management while the child is younger, the upheaval may be less when puberty strikes.

School Lunch

Children with diabetes eat school lunches, just like other kids. Sometimes they like it, and sometimes they don't, just like other kids. School lunches can also present some problems unique to diabetes management. Parents have found a variety of ways to manage the difficulties, with varying levels of cooperation or action from the school. The basic approach is to review the menus with your child, selecting the days when school lunch will be acceptable to the child and reasonably in tune with diabetes management. Most parents seem to use a combination of fine-tuning the insulin doses to handle the actual portions that are provided and working with the child to apply some additional portion control after the tray is delivered. This is obviously more realistic with older school-age kids than with very young ones. Any needed modifications are worked out while the parent and child review the menus. One mom we work with had isolated three school lunch meals that always seemed to send her son's blood sugar too high: spaghetti, pizza, and chicken stir-fry. Talking through the whole selection of things that were served with each of these meals, she and her son were able to agree on some changes he could make on-site: not eat the garlic bread with the spaghetti, eat only two of the three pizza slices, and leave at least half a cup of the rice uneaten on the plate when he had the stir-fry. The youngster preferred doing this to being singled out to get different foods or portions than his friends did.

Some parents tell us they've been able to convince lunchroom personnel to standardize their child's servings to exchange-size (or calorie point or whatever system) portions. This is a matter of the parents' style, how the child feels about the extra attention, and the willingness of the school staff to go along.

Reviewing the menus and finding some way to monitor portion sizes for consistency are necessary, but not sufficient, to ensure that lunch at school will go smoothly. One possible problem that can come up—unscheduled food substitutions—is described at the beginning of the chapter. Another cause of difficulties is odd lunch schedules. This doesn't seem to be an issue everywhere, but in some localities it's quite a hassle, usually beginning in middle school. Kids' lunch periods may be scheduled as early as 10:30 A.M. or as late as 1:30 P.M. For a child on morning NPH or Lente, these kinds of odd schedules can create quite a challenge. For example, one 12-year-old seventh grader who took his morning Regular and NPH before breakfast at about 7:45 A.M. was assigned to the 10:45 A.M. lunch period: just too early to be eating a big lunch in relation to his old insulin regimen. Using the time block approach described in Chapter 4, he and his parents were able to get his morning Regular to cover his breakfast and lunch. Lunch turned out to be nothing much more than a heavy snack, since Todd really wasn't hungry enough to eat a full lunch at 10:45 A.M. anyway. He ate a sandwich at his desk at around 12:15 P.M. and another snack after school when he got home at 3 P.M.

When lunch periods are scheduled too late in relation to the morning insulin injection, a couple of options are possible. A snack containing carbohydrate, protein, and fat (a sandwich, for example) can be eaten at the old normal lunchtime to tide the child over until the late lunch period. Alternatively, the morning NPH or Lente insulin dose can be reduced so it functions more like a background insulin, and an injection of Regular can be taken at the time of the late lunch. Obviously, for this approach to work, the child must be willing and able to take the extra injection at school. This can be made much simpler by using an insulin pen rather than a syringe and vial.

Diabetes Care at School

Making sure that your child's diabetes is managed appropriately at school is obviously very important to your peace of mind and to her well-being. Your child's teachers, principal, school nurse (if you're still lucky enough to have one!), school secretary, food service personnel, and bus driver need some level of diabetes knowledge to ensure her safety. Some of the topics that are helpful to touch on are listed in Table 11.1. You may want to do the honors, your child might, or you might do it together. Guidelines and literature to help you with this important task are available from the American Diabetes Association. In addition, many chapters of the American Association of Diabetes Educators can provide training programs conducted by certified diabetes educators for school personnel. A meeting with all the relevant school staff at the beginning of the year makes sense if you can get cooperation from the school and the individuals involved.

TABLE 11.1 Information Needed by School Personnel

- What diabetes is and isn't (contagious!)
- Care that may/must be done at school
- Low blood glucose (only emergency likely to happen at school)
  Causes
  Symptoms
  Treatment
  What to do if the child refuses to eat
- High blood sugar
  Child's need to drink and go to bathroom
  When to call the parents
- Meals/school lunch
- Snacks
  What
  When
  How you'll provide them
- Gym class
- Parties
- On the bus
- After-school punishment
- Informing substitute teachers

Some words of caution: Don't try to make school personnel into "diabetes police," expecting them to control what your child eats or report to you the specific details of each day. They probably don't have the time, and your child almost certainly won't appreciate being singled out in that way. Obviously, school personnel should be asked to inform you of anything unusual that happens, but being a member of the diabetes police is not part of the cafeteria lady's job description.

Virtually every family struggles with how much testing will be done at school. Before lunch and before gym class are desirable test times, but not everyone can manage to get them done. Testing when low blood sugar is suspected is always a priority. For a child who's too young to do a test independently, it's always more of a challenge. Who will help her, and when and where are they available to take on this extra task? It's also important to determine how your child feels about testing at school before actually deciding what to ask for. In some schools and with some kids, testing is not much of a hassle. Materials are kept in the classroom, and the child and the teacher work out an acceptable and nondisruptive routine. But there's no doubt that in some schools and with some kids, it is a tremendous hassle because of school policies or the individual teachers or other staff members involved. At some schools, for example, testing materials must be kept in the counselor's or nurse's office. In this situation, testing requires pulling the child out of the class's routine and making the test more visible and more disruptive (not to mention risky, if the child is low). If your child must go to a different location to test at school, secure the teacher's agreement to send a companion with her when she's feeling low.

Parties

There are many ways to successfully manage parties, whether they're at school, at a friend's house, or in your own home. There's the "control the environment" school of thought in which parents try to see to it that "offending" foods, such as sweets, are simply not available. This is neither an easy nor a popular approach, and we think it delays the child learning how to make special-occasion foods a controlled part of her life with diabetes. Another strategy is to feed oatmeal or lentils (high in soluble fiber) at breakfast to blunt the effect of eating sweets at school parties. This seems to work best if the party happens during the morning hours. Another possibility is adjusting the insulin upward, after negotiating beforehand the type and amount of extra food she will be eating at the party.

Overnight Stays With Friends

Depending on parental comfort level, having the sleep-overs at your house may be the perfect answer, especially at younger ages. Besides making you very popular with the other parents, this is about the easiest way to give you and your child what you want. You get several things important to your peace of mind: 1) no surprises in the food category, 2) easy observation of how things are going, 3) an opportunity to see what happens to appetite and blood sugar when 8-year-olds stay awake giggling all night, and 4) assurance that neither bedtime nor morning insulin will be forgotten in the shuffle. Your child gets to enjoy her friends' company with your full support.

After doing this a few times, you and your child will have a good idea of what it takes to handle a sleep-over. It will be much easier to make preparations for that first sleep-over at someone else's house, when the time comes. Obviously, the agreement of the hosting parent is very important. Ideally, it will be a parent who already has some experience dealing with your child's needs regarding food, schedules, testing, etc., on shorter visits. But this may not be possible. Several parents we know are true children of the electronic age. They use cellular phones and beepers to ensure everyone's comfort and safety when their child with diabetes is away for longer periods or doing less familiar activities. With this electronic safety net, easy communication is available when questions or problems arise.

Fast food may not be quite as unavoidable as death and taxes, but it's a close call.

• • • •

Fast Food

Fast foods are a familiar feature of the eating landscape for most families and children—as common and expected as pine trees in the forest. They're convenient, relatively inexpensive, tasty, and—probably most important—highly and expertly advertised. The nutritionally dedicated deplore them. Their antagonism may relate to depletion of the rain forest to make grazing room for all those ill-fated cattle or to fast foods' generally high content of fat and sodium. In spite of these and other concerns, most Americans eat at franchise food chains at least twice a week, and the average is even higher for children. Fast food may not be quite as unavoidable as death and taxes, but it's a close call. The wise man recognizes the things he cannot change and learns to deal with them. And so, we accept the inevitability of fast foods! The trick is to know and compensate for their shortcomings while capitalizing on their main benefit for diabetes management. Yes, there actually is a benefit. But, first, those well-recognized shortcomings.

Many fast foods are high in fat and salt, although some lower fat choices are available at most of the larger chains. Choose grilled meat sandwiches instead of the fried ones. Stick with the plainer burgers instead of the double-meat, double-cheese varieties. At McDonald's, you can get a chicken or chef salad with low-fat dressing, and at Wendy's you can choose a bowl of chili, but these are not likely to be high on the hit parade with younger kids. At Taco Bell, there are low-fat versions of several items.

Fat can really add up when a whole meal is chosen off the fast-food menu, especially if the larger sandwiches and fries are included. Fat and salt can be minimized through either item choice or portion size. For example, a burger, fries, and diet soda is a pretty standard fast-food meal or snack. Combining the burger with a side salad with low-fat dressing instead of fries, will greatly reduce the fat and salt content of the meal. However, it's probably more realistic for kids to simply choose the regular size fries instead of the super size. Eliminating or choosing a smaller serving of fries will also provide less carbohydrate compared with eating a large box of fries. If the larger amount of carbohydrate is needed, eating a piece of fruit brought from home can take care of it while also providing a few stray vitamins and minerals. If your child eats fast food frequently, it's worth making these adjustments as a routine matter. If fast foods are an occasional treat, it probably makes more sense to let her eat her favorites with her friends and thus avoid being different. Limiting fat and salt are not really necessary in the short term for most kids, unless they already have blood pressure or blood fat problems. However, since this is the time when lifelong food habits and preferences are being set, it's probably best to encourage lower fat and lower salt intake most of the time. The exchange values and carbohydrate, fat, and sodium content of most fast foods are readily available in literature produced by all the major chains. And that leads to the benefit that fast foods can bring to diabetes management.

For all their shortcomings, fast foods have one enormous advantage when it comes to diabetes control: their consistency. Talk about portion control. Franchise food operations are generally obsessive about portion sizes. Say you sell a couple of million bean burritos a year. If everybody gets an extra ounce of beans on their burrito, it cuts way into your profit margin. That's the main reason employees are trained to make each item consistently. Once you and your child figure out how to fit a given fast-food item into the management plan—either through substitution for other foods in a set meal plan or by adjusting insulin doses appropriately—you're set. Fast food is simply not a wild card anymore, like the lasagna or cookies at a friend's house, where ingredients and portion sizes are often unknowable.

Kid-Style Diabetes Education

If your child was diagnosed at a younger age, any diabetes education that took place was appropriately directed at you. Now that she's reached school age, however, she's old enough to benefit from diabetes education on her own. It should be suited to her age and interest. The right type of diabetes education can be extremely positive. This is the age when, in general, children are very eager to learn about their world and master the skills required for living in it successfully. Knowing more about their diabetes can give them a greater sense of mastery, reducing stress and improving their comfort level.

THE BOTTOM LINE

1. Preschool and school-age children grow up and away from constant parental supervision.
2. A major focus during these years must be helping children learn to control their own blood sugars. This includes learning to choose from a wider variety of foods and doing sufficient blood glucose testing to see the effect.
3. There is an increased need to inform other people about the child's diabetes.
4. Preschoolers are eager to please, which is a great help to your being able to shape more desirable eating habits.
5. Structured meals and snacks help control appetite and promote diabetes control.
6. Review school lunch menus with your child when they are published. Decide when she will get school lunch and, if necessary, how she will modify it.
7. Work with school personnel to ensure that diabetes care gets the appropriate type and amount of attention. Educate and negotiate.
8. Diabetes needn't stop your child from enjoying the same activities as her friends. Parties, overnight stays with buddies, and eating out at fast-food places can all be managed without sacrificing diabetes control.

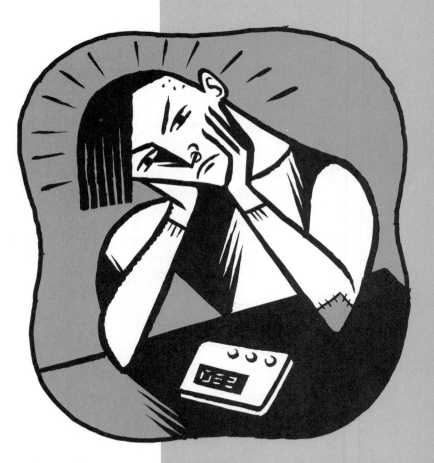

"I keep taking more and more insulin, but my blood sugars aren't getting any better. Mom and Dad think I'm cheating like crazy, and we fight about it a lot."

Teenagers

Adam had been a fixture at diabetes camp every summer since his diabetes was diagnosed at the age of 8. He was a very bright kid, at home with all the diabetes routines, and he had a sweet, quiet way that won him a great many friends. At 13, he seemed like a natural choice to become a Junior Counselor. But when he arrived for the first day of camp, we wondered if we'd made a mistake. In the year since we'd last seen him, Adam's light brown sporty haircut had been replaced by a short, layered cap of jet black hair. Black jacket, clunky walking boots, and sweatshirt matched his inky hair; baggy shorts and a small silver nose ring completed the startling makeover. He definitely had blossomed into full adolescence. Some of the staff wondered out loud if he would be a good influence on the younger campers. We shouldn't have worried.

Under the unique costume was the same sweet Adam. The littlest kids barely seemed to notice his appearance and followed him around in a sort of flying wedge. The older ones pronounced his nose ring either "cool!" or "gross!," and then everyone got on with the business of having a good time. But besides his appearance, something else about Adam had changed since the previous year. His diabetes control had exploded right along with his surging adolescent hormones. This smart kid who seemed to have such a lock on his diabetes self-care the previous summer was now struggling mightily and with little success to contain his soaring blood sugars. He admitted he was immensely relieved to be at camp. There he could escape, at least for awhile, the hassles over diabetes that were raging between him and his parents.

"I know I'm not always as careful as I used to be, but I swear I'm not being this bad," he complained as he tossed his blood glucose record book to the nurse. "My parents are sure it's something I'm doing that's got things so messed up. I wonder if it would actually be any worse if I just blew it all off...my meal plan and testing, I mean. I don't even want to write down my numbers anymore, because I know what's going to happen when Mom and Dad see them."

GROWTH, HORMONES, AND DIABETES CONTROL

Adolescence is a time of huge changes, both emotional and physical. Living through those changes with any youngster is enough challenge for most mere mortals, but things are even more of a struggle when your teen has diabetes. Phenomenal growth and raging hormones often have a huge impact on diabetes control. Adam and his frustrated parents were right in the middle of it. Rising levels of several hormones—especially growth hormone—work against insulin, making it less effective. Glucose control gets harder and harder to achieve as the need for insulin increases. We used to think poor control during the teen years was exclusively the result of a lack of self-care. We now know that's only part of the story. Nature is working mightily against control in growing teens. Keep this in mind the next time you're tempted to raise a major fuss over your teenager's blood sugar results. Insulin requirements remain high while your teen is growing—twice the previous dose is not unusual. Doses will fall back to a more normal level once growth is complete.

EMOTIONAL CHANGE AND DEVELOPMENT

At the very time all this is happening, the emotional changes of adolescence—boundary-testing, risk-taking, identity-seeking—often mean that structured treatment plans are ignored. It's understandable that many parents react to the loss of blood glucose control and the teen's provocative behavior by being more directive. Unfortunately, this generally makes the teen dig in his heels more firmly. The stage is set for escalating arguments over diabetes management. Family relationships take a beating and everybody loses.

Every teen must learn who he is and gain independence. In fact, these are the main tasks of this stage of his life. As important and predictable as it is, however, a teenager's efforts to master these tasks often places diabetes care at risk. This is especially likely if parents respond by going to extremes: either trying to retain control of diabetes management themselves or handing all the responsibility to the teenager. The first extreme is impossible to maintain; no adolescent will tolerate his parents' efforts to manage his diabetes. The second extreme is also fraught with peril; important self-care tasks may fall through the cracks, because few teens are prepared to fly solo when it comes to diabetes care.

The trick is to stay involved without being overbearing. Blood sugar control—and everyone's sanity and comfort—will be better if responsibility for diabetes management is gradually shifted from parent to teen, with parents always continuing to participate in their teen's diabetes care in some supportive, mutually agreed upon way. Try to look on mistakes as learning opportunities. Ask lots of questions that help your teen think through what happened. Get him to talk about how he was affected by the outcome. Ask him how he might use what he learned in the future to produce a better outcome.

And don't criticize what he eats! Doing so only hands him a script for getting your goat. Remember, teens need to test boundaries. Don't wave unnecessary red flags in front of your teen's face. He's likely to charge. Teenagers who are criticized about their eating habits skip more meals and have worse overall eating habits than teens whose families take a more relaxed and philosophical attitude. By philosophical we mean 1) accepting the fact that blood sugar goals should probably be less strict during adolescence, especially during growth spurts and when cooperation is more problematic, and 2) understanding that adolescence is a self-limiting condition. In other words, it will end. If you and your child are still friends when he comes out of the tunnel of adolescence and you have managed to avoid major problems with his diabetes, you all deserve a huge pat on the back.

THE TIME FOR INDEPENDENT DOCTOR VISITS

This can be a good time for him to start seeing the doctor and educator on his own. This doesn't mean that you should totally give up your involvement. It's another case of finding a middle road that meets both your needs. You will still want to have at least occasional joint visits with the health-care team. Or you may want to go to every visit together, with some time included for your kid to spend alone with the health-care provider. Independent medical visits will be welcomed by most teens, but the main reason to accept or even encourage them is that they provide your teen with some privacy. This is important, because a bit of privacy may encourage more frank communication pertaining to touchy adolescent subjects, such as sex and drinking. Handling a medical visit on his own also signals your trust in his developing ability to take care of his own diabetes. And it's an important step in his learning to establish an independent relationship with his health-care provider. It's best that he begin to practice his skills for communicating with health-care providers while you are still available to discuss how it's going and provide guidance as appropriate. A summary report on the visit—excluding any confidential information—prepared by the doctor or educator can help keep parents engaged, while still giving the teen the desired increase in privacy and independence.

THE IMPORTANCE OF PEER RELATIONSHIPS

This is the age where relationships with peers become the major focus of most kids' lives. Even family ties sometimes may take a backseat to friendships. At times, teens seem to have only two goals: to be as different from their parents as possible and to be as much like their friends as possible. Because his friends are so important, your child probably wants to do whatever they are doing. This helps him feel comfortable and secure. If his friends dress all in black and read old beatnik poetry, you may find it irritating, but it doesn't really affect diabetes care (or anything else important, either). On the other hand, if the friends spend a lot of time hanging around the mall eating after school, your teen with diabetes will probably do the same, and the impact on diabetes control will be substantial. Take our word for it. It is more productive to work with him to help him find ways to reduce the diabetes fallout from such activities than it is to keep screaming, "Look at your blood sugar! You shouldn't do that!!"

Making an issue of these things, especially in a way that your teen feels is critical or nagging, usually escalates the confrontation. Whether the resulting disagreement is played out as a multi-decibel donnybrook or in stony silence, chances are that you still won't get what you want. In fact, diabetes self-care and control may get worse. When you throw down the gauntlet over some aspect of self-care, in effect, you hand your teen a perfect tool for resisting your authority: bona fide and guaranteed effective. Remember that resisting authority is an essential part of every teenager's job description. Try to keep diabetes care out of the fray as much as possible. You do this by not criticizing his self-care efforts, even when sorely tempted. Instead, use the questioning and problem-solving approach described in Chapter 5.

Over the years, one of us has made the following deal with many teens who were struggling against their parents and their diabetes: "If you're looking for a way to get your parents' goat, look someplace other than your diabetes. Pierce your nose. Dye your hair blue. Do whatever your friends are doing. But promise me you won't skip your insulin. That's just too risky." This worked very well for many years. Inevitably though, one day the call came in from an irate father. "My son says he dyed his hair blue because you told him he could! What have you got to say for yourself?" That one took some explaining!

ERRATIC SCHEDULES

Stable schedules aren't part of most teenagers' lives. After-school activities mean many kids don't come home at all in the afternoon. If your teen has that kind of schedule, the days of laying out the after-school snack and being able to count on its time and composition are gone. Snacks may be coming from different sources and at different times on different days of the week.

Gina's schedule was one of those. Her mother's happiest day came when Gina got her driver's license. It marked the day Mom could stop transporting the busy high school junior to all of her various activities. On Monday, Gina grabbed a small hamburger and a diet soda at a fast-food drive-through window on her way to ballet class after school. On Tuesday afternoon, she stayed on campus for cheerleading practice. She had to remember to bring something from home because the snack bar was closed after school. On Wednesday afternoon, she needed less of a snack because she was working on the yearbook. That one had to be brought from home, too, and she ate it a little later. Thursday, she went home after school and could fix her own snack when she got there. What she ate varied depending on whether she was going to stay home and study or head back out to do something more active with her friends. Friday night, she usually had a ball game of some sort to attend. She needed to make sure that her snack and her dinner were pretty substantial, since the cheerleading she did at the games really dropped her blood sugar. It was another fast-food night, as a rule.

STAYING UP ALL NIGHT AND SLEEPING LATE

One of the schedule problems that usually surfaces during adolescence involves late nights and the even later mornings that often follow them. Staying up late by itself does not have a large effect on insulin needs or diabetes control. The teen who stays up all night studying, reading, or watching TV may not see much of a difference in his blood sugar. Naturally, the story would be different if late nights also meant extra snacking without extra insulin to compensate for it. But when a teen is staying out late doing more, the effect on control can be dramatic. To complicate matters, a teenager may be out dancing (lowers blood sugar), eating extra food (raises blood sugar), and drinking alcohol (increases risk for low blood sugar), all in the same evening. The only reasonable way to approach these situations is with an inquiring mind and a lot of blood glucose test strips. Testing before and after going out provides the information you and your teen will need to start identifying patterns. Of course, the more details you know (how much dancing, what kind of food, how many beers, and so on), the more meaningful the blood glucose results will be. Past history can be a great help to choosing reasonable management options, but only if enough information was gathered previously.

The child who wants to sleep late—a favorite teen pastime—has a challenge. Sleeping through the usual morning injection may mean running out of insulin and waking up with very high blood sugar. Waking up briefly to take a shot without eating breakfast puts him at high risk for low blood sugar. Does that mean he has to abandon his hopes of having a lazy morning in the sack? No. There are several options for reconciling sleeping late with reasonable diabetes control. As is the case with many things in life, the easiest one is also the most expensive! Get an insulin pump. When the basal rate on a pump is set correctly, sleeping late and skipping meals is not a management problem. Blood sugars stay stable while the teen snoozes. When he gets up, he takes a premeal dose of Regular insulin through the pump to handle breakfast (or lunch) when he actually eats it. None of the options open to those who aren't on the pump work quite so neatly, but they still get the job done. There are a couple of inescapable facts that must be considered as you work out the best plan. One is that insulin must be taken reasonably close to the prescribed time. If it isn't, the liver will start releasing glucose during sleep, and the first blood sugar of the day will be sky high. There may be urine ketones as well, because the teen has run out of insulin by delaying the shot too long. The other given is that you can't wake up in the morning, take your usual insulin dose, and then go back to sleep without eating. The most likely result of that choice would be a low blood sugar reaction.

This is a perfect example of a situation where asking questions and trying experiments can help you and your teen work out an acceptable solution. Options to consider include reversing the order of the morning snack and the breakfast, with the snack eaten after the injection and before returning to bed for that last delicious hour or two of sleep. The full breakfast can then be eaten at mid-morning. Another possibility is to go with a really simple substitution for the usual breakfast. Say a good-sized muffin and a glass of milk. Another option for the late sleeper is to take the NPH, Lente, or Ultralente insulin at the normal time and hold the Regular insulin until later when the meal will be eaten. You could also consider splitting the morning Regular insulin dose, taking only one or two units at the usual time to tide the youngster over the remaining hour or two of sleep. (This is probably needed if the overnight insulin is predinner NPH or Lente.) The remainder of the morning Regular can be taken when he actually gets up and eats breakfast. Another option is to move predinner NPH or Lente to bedtime so that it will better cover the next morning. Probably the simplest approach of all for teens who have this need, and other needs for flexible timing, is Ultralente in the morning and evening, with Regular insulin given at mealtime. The specific approach you settle on is a matter of personal choice and the blood glucose results that you find. Experimentation will tell you and your teen which approach has the best combination of effectiveness and acceptability.

TEEN APPETITES AND CALORIE NEEDS

Many teenagers have huge appetites. Most adults would consider a hamburger, fries, and a diet soda a reasonably sized meal. The teen appetite may demand twice that amount for an after-school snack. Kids will almost surely eat what and when their friends do. If substantial after-school snacks are part of your child's routine and they are interfering with good blood sugar control, you have a problem that needs solving. You and your teen need to explore approaches that will give both of you what you want. Perhaps he wants to have fast food after school like everybody else. You want his blood sugar to be somewhere near the planet Earth by the time dinner rolls around. There may be fast-food choices that will minimize the rise in blood glucose. Or, it may be possible to increase the morning NPH insulin to provide better coverage. The downside of this approach is that it locks him into eating a large amount every day. An additional small bolus of Regular insulin taken only on the days when he goes out for fast food with his friends might be a reasonable and acceptable way to keep blood sugars in check. This would be easier to do using an insulin pen. Remember, if your child didn't have diabetes and was eating that amount of food, his body would be putting out extra insulin to metabolize it.

Because calorie needs can be so large at this age, enormous meals may not be associated with any unwanted weight gain. This is most likely if the teen is large, growing, physically active, and male. All of these factors greatly increase energy needs. A 17-year-old girl who has stopped growing probably would have much lower calorie needs than a 17-year-old boy of similar size. The difference in young men, compared with young women, relates to the boys' generally larger muscle mass. Muscles use more calories per pound than other types of body tissue.

The amount of food that it takes to meet most teens' nutrient needs (for protein, vitamins, minerals, and so on) is much less than the amount of food it takes to meet their energy needs. Therefore, they can afford empty calories to a greater extent than most younger children or adults. That's why most teens can eat potato chips, cheese curls, french fries, chili, pizza, cookies, and ice cream—all those things that provide relatively little nutrition for their large calorie cost—without gaining weight or developing some dreaded nutritional deficiency disease. Not that these foods, with their high fat content, are exactly the stuff of a dietitian's dreams, of course. But they are a reality of many teens' diets, and they can be consumed without any known bad effects during those times when calorie needs are high.

If you're worried that your child is eating too much, remember the discussion from Chapter 2 about how to tell if your child is eating the right amount of food. If weight is staying normal and diabetes control is reasonable, chances are that the amount of food is just what your child needs to fuel the current growth spurt. But remember also that a child with diabetes may lose or maintain weight, even if he's eating more than he needs, if control is quite poor. When control is poor, sugar and all the calories it contains leave the body in large quantities, creating a large calorie drain. On the other hand, if a child eats more than he needs and successfully chases all that extra food with insulin to keep blood sugar in check, he will gain weight, just like people who don't have diabetes. If you are concerned about eating problems and eating disorders, see Chapter 9.

ALCOHOL, DRIVING, TOBACCO, DRUGS, AND SEX

Experimenting with alcohol, drugs, and sex is extremely common in teens. Statistics tell us that the children who engage in one or more of these behaviors, at least occasionally, greatly outnumber those who don't. We might wish that this wasn't so, but it is. It's important to face the realities. If you can manage to discuss these topics in a reasonably comfortable and nonaccusing fashion, talk to your teen. If you can't be objective about it, make sure another responsible adult does it.

Alcohol. Pure alcohol does not raise blood glucose. The body handles alcohol very much like fat. That's why some health-care providers recommend that people with diabetes exchange alcohol for fat in the meal plan. We don't recommend exchanging alcohol for a couple of reasons. First, if a teen is going to drink alcohol (which is not only illegal but probably discouraged by his parents), we don't think he's going to bother counting exchanges while he's doing it. Furthermore, it's not necessary. Pure alcohol has no effect on blood sugar, so people with type I diabetes can just add modest amounts of alcohol to their food intake without raising blood sugar. By "modest" we mean up to two drinks, if a drink is understood to be a 12-ounce beer, a glass of wine, or an ounce of distilled liquor.

More alcohol than this won't raise blood sugar directly, but it's still likely to have an effect on blood sugar. People who are drinking larger amounts of alcohol tend to ignore their self-care. They are less aware of what they're eating, they may forget to take insulin on time, and so on. Also, because alcohol raises the risk for hypoglycemia, heavier drinking gets quite risky.

While the body is processing alcohol, it is unable to release sugar from the liver, even if the blood sugar level gets dangerously low. In addition, alcohol increases the efficiency of whatever insulin is already in the body. Someone with type I diabetes who is drinking is not only more likely to have a low blood sugar reaction but also more likely to have a severe reaction, because the body is not able to respond normally to the falling glucose level.

Unless someone actually gives a teen the facts about alcohol and diabetes, he is likely to make some dangerous assumptions. We have encountered a lot of youngsters who viewed sweets and alcohol as very similar, because they had been told at some point to stay away from both. A teen working without accurate information may skip a meal when he's experimenting with alcohol. It seems like a logical way to exchange if you don't know the real effects of alcohol. He ends up putting himself at great risk for hypoglycemia. Since drinking is a distinct possibility from at least junior high school on, kids from about the age of 12 need to have the straight scoop on alcohol. In addition to the facts about hypoglycemia risk described here and in Chapter 7, teens should know at least the following guidelines:

- If you're going to drink, keep the amounts small. Up to two drinks can be added to the normal meal pattern with relatively little effect on blood sugar.
- Because of the risk for low blood sugar, never skip meals when drinking alcohol.
- Choose light beers, dry wines, or distilled liquor, and use non-caloric mixers. If sweet drinks and mixers are

used, their carbohydrate must be taken into account. The carbohydrate in sweeter drinks may raise blood sugar. Insulin can be adjusted to compensate for this, but it can get complicated when paired with the hypoglycemic effect of the alcohol itself.

- Wear a diabetes medical I.D. at all times, but especially when drinking. Others (friends, police) might confuse low blood sugar for drunkenness if you've been drinking.
- Make sure someone in your group knows about your diabetes and what to do about low blood sugar. This is always important, but even more so if you're drinking alcohol.

Driving. Getting a driver's license marks a big day in every teen's life. It's a double-antacid day for most parents, however. It's hard to feel confident about your 16-year-old maneuvering several tons of steel through busy streets. You remember him running over flower beds on his bike because his steering wasn't the best. You've seen him walk into walls because he wasn't watching where he was going. When the teen in question has diabetes, the stresses that surround driving are multiplied. In addition to all the usual concerns that accompany any teen's foray onto the highway, the teen with diabetes has hypo-glycemia risk to consider. And the risk is real. Blood sugars can drop when your child is behind the wheel just as they can at any other time. The potential for trouble is just greater. The teenager is now in a position to seriously harm both himself and others if his blood sugar drops low enough to slow his thinking or responses. And of course, drinking and driving is an especially dangerous combination for the teen with diabetes.

This is one of those areas that cry out for good communication, questioning, and problem-solving. Teens want to drive. Parents want them to be safe. Mutually acceptable guidelines for eating, drinking, testing, and driving are needed if both sets of desires are going to be fulfilled.

Tobacco. Once started, smoking and chewing tobacco are very hard habits to break, and their potential for harm grows the longer they're maintained. While they have little or no effect on blood glucose control per se, they do impair circulation in the short run. In the long run, they are harmful to blood vessels and greatly increase cancer risk. But these health risks rarely discourage people from tobacco use. Some teens try smoking or chewing because everybody else is doing it, or because it makes them feel grown up. It's hard to sell kids on a long-term issue like cancer risk or an old people's problem like heart disease. But teens who smoke or chew need to know the risks. Keep in mind, however, that they may actually be more impressed with a couple of negative outcomes from smoking and chewing that are of more immediate concern in their world. Tobacco makes you smell and taste bad: a pretty good argument with teens who are interested in being attractive. Although they can get around that one by finding a boyfriend or girlfriend who also smokes. Kids who are physically active may also be concerned that smoking reduces stamina. It's hard to run the 440 when you're coughing your head off!

Drugs. Many prescription and over-the-counter drugs have effects that are important to consider in managing diabetes. For example, drugs may lower blood glucose, raise blood glucose, affect heart rate, interfere with sexual function, or upset the stomach. If your child with diabetes takes a prescription or over-the-counter drug, ask your pharmacist if it has any diabetes-specific effects.

Illegal drugs. Recreational drugs—also called drugs of abuse—have many potential negative effects, some of which are specific to blood sugar control. We will touch on just two of them here: marijuana and cocaine. These two drugs have specific appetite effects that have implications for diabetes management. Marijuana is notorious for bringing on the munchies or uncontrolled eating binges. Just about anything edible seems to be fair game, but sweets are particularly attractive. Marijuana munchies can lead to pretty outrageous disturbances in diabetes control. Someone high on pot is probably not thinking clearly enough to calculate the supplemental insulin dose for a whole bag of chocolate chip cookies! In fact, one of the most profound ways in which all forms of substance abuse affect diabetes management relates to the altered states they produce. Being drunk or high usually leads to abandonment of basic self-care practices. The test doesn't get done. The meal gets skipped. The dose of insulin is forgotten or taken incorrectly.

Quite the opposite of marijuana, cocaine may reduce appetite and contribute to weight loss. This is, in fact, one of its attractions for some people. Cocaine acts like epinephrine (adrenaline). Because of this, it may raise blood glucose in spite of the reduction in appetite and food intake it usually causes. Of course, these and other drugs of abuse have many other negative effects. If you suspect your teen is using drugs, blood glucose control is only one of your concerns. We encourage you to get the information and support you both need to deal with this serious problem. Your pharmacist, physician, or diabetes educator are all good resources.

Sex. And speaking of subjects that are difficult to discuss calmly with your teenager! As much as parents wish that teens would abstain from sex until they're older (for a wide variety of moral, ethical, and practical reasons), the fact remains that many teens are sexually active. For the teen with diabetes and his parents, sex has many of the same features as driving a car. First, it is an activity with its own set of significant risks that the teen with diabetes shares with all other teens. In the case of sex, those risks are huge: AIDS, other sexually transmitted diseases, and pregnancy, just for starters. Since unprotected sex with the wrong person could literally cost a teen his life in the era of AIDS, many realistic parents have seen to it that their child has condoms . . . just in case.

And, as is the case with driving, diabetes adds additional risks of its own. One diabetes-specific risk is relatively mild: hypoglycemia. Like any type of physical exertion, sex can produce hypoglycemia. The embarrassment factor is probably at least as big an issue as the risk from the low blood sugar itself. Risk for hypoglycemia during or after sexual intercourse is greater if blood sugar is on the low side to begin with and if insulin levels are fairly high. Prevention and treatment are the same as for any form of physical activity. The reality, of course, is that few teens will have the forethought and self-confidence to test blood sugar and stop for a snack before (or while) having sex. Maybe there ought to be a tube of glucose gel with the condoms...just in case.

The other diabetes-specific risk of sex is far more serious: potential bad outcomes of pregnancy for the baby of a mom with diabetes. Of course, teen pregnancy has huge implications for everyone concerned: the young mother and father, the baby, the grandparents, and the society. If the pregnant teen has diabetes, the problems and risks may be greatly multiplied. When pregnancy in diabetes is expertly managed, the health of the baby and the mother are no different than for any other pregnancy. But—and it's a very big "but"—for that to occur, diabetes control has to be excellent before conception. The pregnancy must be planned. This is rarely the case when a teen becomes pregnant outside of marriage. If the mother's glucose control is not good when she conceives, the baby is at significant risk for birth defects. If you add an impaired baby to the load created by a teen pregnancy, the potential burden is enormous.

Prevention is by far the best course. Talk this over with your teenage daughter. If sexual activity is a possibility (or a reality), you or she need to discuss contraception options with her health-care team. Birth control pills are the most reliable form of contraception, and they can be used by women with diabetes. Obviously, pills alone don't confer any protection against AIDS and other sexually transmitted diseases. The only totally safe option is abstinence, but skillful condom use greatly reduces the risk for disease transmission when compared with unprotected sex. Together, pills and condoms provide the greatest possible protection against pregnancy and sexually transmitted diseases.

The nutritional needs of a pregnant teen with diabetes are quite impressive. Pregnancy itself increases the need for calories, protein, folic acid, iron, and several other nutrients. When those needs are superimposed on the high energy and nutrient demands created by teenage growth and development, the nutritional stakes get pretty high. Finally, add the complexity of balancing nutritional intake with insulin to produce stellar glucose control. Now you have a major production on your hands. A pregnant teen with diabetes needs to be working with a skillful dietitian or other diabetes educator to help her with this complex task. An endocrinologist (to manage the diabetes) and a skilled obstetrician/gynecologist (to follow the pregnancy) are also needed.

HELPING YOUR TEEN IDENTIFY HIS MOTIVATION FOR BETTER CONTROL

Diabetes control during the teen years is a huge challenge. If a teen doesn't get something he values highly out of better control, the chance of him doing all those hard self-care tasks is really small. The risk of long-term complications just doesn't impress most teens. They live in the here and now. Twenty years into the future doesn't seem real to them. Adolescents also have a general feeling of invincibility—bad things may happen to other people but not to them. They may understand the risks intellectually but simply not feel personally vulnerable. Motivators, to be powerful, need to be more immediate: feeling your best, being able to participate in sports, avoiding hypoglycemia and the embarrassment and disruption it can cause.

One of the best arguments for better control that we have found—especially for boys—is the fact that poor control places muscle mass and growth at risk. Most young men want to reach their full growth potential. And most are also interested in being strong and having good muscle mass. Neither of those things happen when diabetes control is poor. Reaching full height also can be an issue for girls. If she spends all her life as a smaller person, her need for calories will be less than if she gained her full height. Because of those lower energy needs, she may need to be more careful about food intake and exercise in order to prevent unwanted weight gain.

Help your teen think through the benefits he may get from better control. Every kid is different. Help your kid find his motivation: his reasons to maintain good control, not yours. Lots of questions and discussion are the best approach we know of to find the answers.

PUMPS OR MULTIPLE INJECTIONS FOR TEENS

Stringent blood glucose goals are not a realistic option for a great many teens. As we've said before, the difficulties of control relate to hormone changes, the rebellious attitudes of some adolescents, and the struggles that many of them have in maintaining regular schedules. These challenges cause many diabetes programs to routinely exclude teens from intensive therapy, but we'd like to make a distinction between stringent goals and the tools of intensive therapy used to achieve them. We feel that some teens benefit greatly from intensive forms of therapy, even if somewhat looser blood glucose goals have been set. We like these treatment options because they provide greater flexibility for adjusting food and insulin to meet actual demands. They can also be a tremendous help for teens who take part in sports or other activities that challenge diabetes management skills. In other words, for any typical teenager.

To achieve glucose control, unchanging insulin doses must be paired with unchanging food intake, exercise routines, and schedules. Teens are, as a group, even less able to maintain that kind of stability and self-discipline than the rest of us. So these tools, such as learning to adjust premeal insulin doses for actual food intake, can be particularly welcome to them.

Pumps provide the greatest flexibility because, when used expertly, they all but erase the time restrictions that are so hard for teens to deal with. With a pump, there's no more necessity to eat a certain amount at a certain time. There's the ability to reduce insulin during exercise—even when you didn't plan to be active hours ahead of time. That greatly reduces the risk for low blood sugars during and after exercise. There's also the ability to sleep late on the weekend without bouncing out of bed to take the morning shot. But there is a downside to all that flexibility.

Having a pump means that the wearer must pay more attention to his diabetes, because pumps require even more self-care routines than other forms of therapy. In addition to everything else, with a pump, you need to check the infusion set every day, change it every couple of days, and be doubly responsible about frequent and regular blood glucose testing. The other downside to a pump that many teens find hard to deal with is its visibility. Depending on how it's worn, it can make your diabetes more obvious—and a source of curiosity—to people around you. Some teens can't deal with someone else seeing them hooked up to it, like in gym class, at the beach, or in more intimate moments. Some teens also object to the pump because it interferes with their body image. Or, the thought of being dependent on a machine may be disturbing in itself.

Many teens and their parents have thought this through, balanced the downside against the benefits, and opted for pump therapy. It's certainly not for everyone, but it has been a successful option for many teens. It makes a bit more room for some of the realities of teen life.

FAMILY MEALS ARE STILL IMPORTANT

In spite of the fact that many teens want to eat all their meals away from home, it's still extremely valuable to keep up the structure of family mealtimes. The more they eat at home, the better their overall nutritional status is likely to be. This is because kids are more likely to drink milk and eat fruits and vegetables at home than at other places. These foods provide important nutrients that tend to be missing from the diets of teens who seldom eat at home.

This is a good time to revisit the parents' job description as it relates to teenagers. The parents' job description remains the same even though your teen is eating fewer and fewer meals with the family.

1. Get the right stuff into the house and onto the table. Include plenty of snack items, since heavy snacking is a very common feature of teen eating. You can greatly improve the quality of what your teen eats by stocking healthy snacks: fruits, bagels, whole-grain breads, lean meats and low-fat cheeses for sandwiches, low-fat or skim milk, yogurt, soup, and cereal. They contribute to

good nutrition and health while filling up that great, gaping, bottomless pit of teenage hunger. High-fat, high-sugar snack foods just fill the pit.

2. Continue to have family meals and expect the kids to be there, even though you know they won't always be. This reinforces the message that regular meals are important. If teens can't be at a family meal because of other commitments, they should let you know. This shows respect for your efforts to prepare meals, and it keeps the teen hooked into the process, even though he's not always participating in it actively.

THE BOTTOM LINE

1. The physical, developmental, and emotional upheavals of adolescence make diabetes control a real challenge. Somewhat less ambitious blood glucose goals may be needed.

2. Parents need to stay involved and avoid criticizing the teen's efforts at self-control.

3. The teen's desire for privacy and the possible emergence of sensitive issues, like sex and alcohol, make this a good time to start independent doctor visits.

4. Teens' erratic schedules call for sophisticated management skills guided by the results of blood glucose testing.

5. Teens need early, accurate education about the effects and risks of alcohol use in diabetes.

6. The interaction of diabetes with driving, sex, and drugs needs frank discussion to keep your teen safe.

7. The tools of intensive therapy—multiple injections or a pump and insulin adjustment for changes in food and activity—can add much-needed flexibility to a teen's management plan. The tools can be used even when less demanding blood glucose goals are being used.

IV SECTION

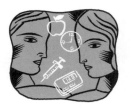

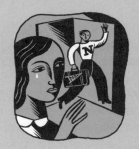

The last section of the book contains some thoughts on how parents can keep their own balance and reason while dealing with all of the demands of managing diabetes and a family.

AND DON'T FORGET TO TAKE CARE OF YOU

The last section of the book contains some thoughts on how parents can keep their own balance and reason while dealing with all of the demands of managing diabetes and a family. In chapter 13, we deal with the comfort and coping of the whole family, but with special emphasis on the needs of Mom and Dad. Chapter 14 describes the most effective ways we know of to support and encourage your child as she learns to care for her own diabetes, because as we've said before, that's the real key to parenting the child with diabetes successfully.

The focus of this book is the nutritional issues that concern your family. After all, good nutrition is very important to overall health and to successful diabetes management. And we give you a lot of ideas throughout the book about how to better manage this vital part of your child's diabetes care. But we can't emphasize strongly enough that, just as nutrition can't be separated from diabetes in your child's life, diabetes can't be controlled in a vacuum. Good diabetes control only happens in families that are coping reasonably well with the same issues of parenting, loving, discipline, and life that concern every other family.

We close with these two chapters to help you keep the nutritional strategies properly placed in the context of a well-functioning, reasonably sane family.

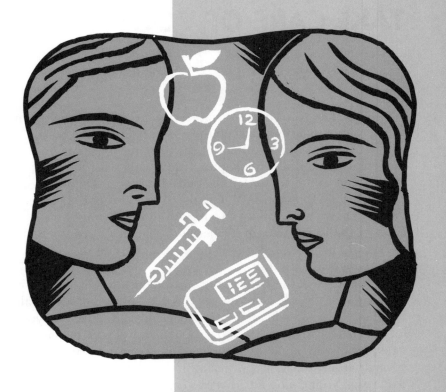

"Lonnie and Dave were buried under the daily management of Trudy's diabetes."

An Action Plan for Avoiding Diabetes Overwhelmus Mom-and-Popus

Sometimes I feel like I've lost my wife, like I'm living with this really intense nurse.

When Dave and Lonnie came to the office, they were like most parents we see for the first time: concerned, loving, tired, and more than a little bit nuts. "We haven't been out together alone since Trudy's had diabetes," Dave told us. "Lonnie's afraid to leave her with a baby-sitter. She does every blood sugar check and insulin shot herself. She makes every meal. She's the one who knows the most about it, so she takes care of it. Sometimes I feel like I've lost my wife, like I'm living with this really intense nurse."

"I just feel better doing it myself," Lonnie countered. "You know I wouldn't enjoy myself if we went out anyway. I'd be too worried that Trudy was home conning the sitter out of stuff she shouldn't eat or running around too much until she had a reaction or something." Lonnie and her husband were suffering from what we might call diabetes overwhelmus mom-and-popus. Don't let the silly name fool you.

This is as big a threat to their daughter's long-term health as the diabetes. And it's common. Every parent of a child with diabetes is affected at one time or another. But when the condition becomes chronic, it spells trouble for the whole family.

Lonnie and Dave were overwhelmed. They were buried under the daily management of Trudy's diabetes. They were stressed and unhappy. Each of them felt frustrated and isolated, and their marriage was suffering. Fun and relaxation had gone on the endangered species list when diabetes appeared on the scene. Trudy's control was quite good when we first saw her family, but all of them were paying a very high price for it. And if Lonnie and Dave are like most parents, they couldn't have kept up the pace indefinitely. Eventually, the stress would have led to arguments, burnout, or both, with bad fallout for the family and the diabetes. Avoiding diabetes overwhelmus is important, not only for the family's current quality of life but also for the long-term picture.

Remember the gorilla at the symphony? In the **Introduction: What Diabetes Can Do To Families,** we talked about how the diabetes gorilla can divert your attention from the important symphony of your child's growth and development. Another big risk of paying all that attention to diabetes is that it makes you forget to take proper care of yourself and your partner. This can be a real problem. If there's one thing that your child with diabetes needs, it's sane, healthy parents who are as happy, relaxed, and secure as possible. You are your child's advocate, protector, and role model. If you get exhausted and frustrated, she will feel the fallout in a negative way—even if you got that way doing things for her welfare!

STAYING SANE AND HEALTHY

Get the whole family involved. We've already mentioned this, but we'd like to repeat it because it's so important. No matter what your child's age, effective diabetes care requires that you, your child with diabetes, and everyone else in the family work together as a team. Your goal is to raise a happy, healthy child with whom you have a strong and loving relationship. You can do it, but only if you make diabetes care a partnership: a cooperative effort among all the members of the family.

Often, Mom ends up doing too much: going to all the medical appointments, taking responsibility for the food, giving all the injections and finger sticks to little kids, and so on. Dad needs to be a part of this, too. And other kids, in age-appropriate ways, of course. Not only does this free up some of Mom's time to work on other family priorities and on keeping her own balance and sanity, but it's also reassuring for the child with diabetes to feel that bigger support system around her. It's generally satisfying for Dad and the other kids, as well. It's real help that's needed, and being truly helpful feels good to us all. We've suggested many techniques to help distribute the diabetes load. One technique is breaking up needed routines into individual tasks and then dividing the tasks up among different family members. Another is asking questions to identify exactly what kind of help the child with diabetes wants from other family members.

Make sure that your blood sugar goals are realistic. Remember, perfect control is impossible to achieve using the medical tools we have available now. This is especially true during your child's teenage years, when a combination of wing testing and hormonal changes often make blood sugar control particularly rocky. Cut your child and yourself a little slack. Agree on "good-enough" goals that keep the child feeling well but keep the self-care burden manageable. You will find it improves both your family life and your child's willingness to work at controlling her diabetes. Don't forget to identify nondiabetes-related goals for yourself and the family, as well. Being clear about what you want out of life makes it much easier to make choices about what you can and will do to get there. Balance the enjoyment and quality of your short-term lifestyle against the long-term concerns, like preventing complications. Remember, diabetes control and family sanity are a package deal. You can't have one without the other.

Get feelings out in the open. At first, some people think that delving into their feelings about dealing with their child's diabetes is not very practical. You already know you worry ...so what? In fact, dealing with emotions is a very practical part of managing both your peace of mind and the diabetes. Living with diabetes simply makes life more stressful. As a result, everyone in the family is bound to feel frustrated, scared, and angry at times. When they do, they need to find a constructive way to let out the feelings. Held inside, unexpressed emotions continue to upset you and to grow. Expressing them may not make them go away, but it allows you to get them out where you can work on them, allowing you to ask for support and help in dealing with them, if necessary.

When tempers flare, it may help to remember that it's most often the diabetes you are upset with, not each other. Maybe this doesn't sound quite right to you at first, but if you think about it, you may find you agree. After all, having diabetes isn't fair. It imposes a lot of hard work and worry on the family. There's plenty to be angry about. It's okay, and probably even necessary, to acknowledge and express that anger. Let it energize the family's work in dealing with the diabetes, instead of turning it on each other. Also, focusing your anger (or other upset feelings) on the diabetes puts you and your child on the same side of the fence. A family united to deal with diabetes can get a lot more done than a family that's constantly blaming each other for the problems related to dealing with it.

If getting things out in the open hasn't been your family's style, you may wonder exactly how to go about it. The best way depends on the specific feeling in question and on your child's age and personality. Young kids often get relief (and a good laugh) when they unleash their anger at diabetes by stomping around the house yelling, "I hate diabetes!" You might find it helpful too. Feel free to join the parade. Your kid will love the fact that 1) you're being a bit silly and 2) you feel like she does. Punching pillows or throwing them against a blank wall is another popular way to vent. (Be careful about throwing a pillow into a corner and kicking it hard. We had one dad who broke a big toe when he got carried away during an I Hate Diabetes Parade.) Less physical youngsters may enjoy drawing angry pictures—smashed syringes, dismantled blood test meters, and the like. Older kids and adults sometimes get relief from simply talking about their hurt, anger, or resentment.

Painful as it may be for you to hear your child express her sad or angry feelings, it's important to let her do it. Pain is a fact of life. It's not unique to diabetes, but diabetes definitely adds to the load. In spite of that reality, parents sometimes feel they can lessen the pain by telling their children that diabetes isn't really so bad, that the child shouldn't feel as she does. In our experience, this only makes matters worse. The child knows how she feels. The parent's efforts to get her to feel otherwise almost always backfire, making her feel bad about herself, cut off from her parents, or both.

Feeling bad about diabetes is natural and normal, maybe even inevitable. When your child expresses these feelings and you acknowledge them, they become less of a problem. Parents can feel powerless when their child talks about how much she hates diabetes, because they don't know what to do about those feelings. They think they should be able to make the pain go away. But it's not possible. Feelings cannot be fixed or made to go away with some simple reassurance. What they need is to be expressed, accepted, and dealt with. The best thing you can do to help that process along, in fact the only helpful thing you can do, is to listen to your child and to love her. It works.

Then there are *your* feelings. You probably sometimes get frustrated, angry, and scared about things your child has done or not done about her diabetes care. You, too, have to let those feelings out. The key to doing this constructively is to talk about how you are feeling, not about what your child is doing. If, for example, your child is having a tough time staying away from some food that sends her blood sugar through the roof, you may be tempted (as anyone might) to get on her case for cheating. But blaming won't change her behavior, and it's almost guaranteed to drive a wedge between you. Instead, try telling her how her behavior makes you feel: scared, frustrated, confused, etc.

This approach probably won't get your child to immediately go back on her nutrition plan either. But you will have found a way to vent your feelings without driving her away. This will help prevent excess anger and resentment from building up over time.

It's possible that your child may respond to your expression of feeling as if you were criticizing her. If this happens, you can tell her that you know you can't control her behavior, although you wish you could. Explain that you are just letting out your feelings. Assure her that when she tells you how she feels, you will do your best to listen to her. Ask her to try to do the same when you let out your feelings. This is not only a valuable release for you, it models for the child more effective ways to deal with her own angry or hurt feelings. It's both reassuring and a bit frightening to remember that our children learn nearly everything from us by example. We talked about this earlier in the context of promoting good nutritional habits. It's equally true with regard to how children learn to deal with emotion and conflict.

Obviously, the extent to which you share your feelings with your child will depend a lot on how old she is. This technique probably is not much use with very young children, though sharing feelings of anger at the diabetes or resentment at the demands and restrictions it imposes works with kids of any age.

Know what's needed medically and ask for it...if necessary, demand it. The American Diabetes Association and others have defined good diabetes care. An excellent way to deal with the fears you have about your child's health is to know what the experts say needs to be done and then double-check that your own team is following through. There are a lot of details in diabetes management. Sometimes, health-care providers get very focused on what is going on today—the immediate problem, like the very low blood sugar that your child had last week—and forget about the long-term picture. If they need reminding, do it.

Here's the minimum: your child should see her doctor at least four times per year for midcourse corrections. This helps make sure that the therapy keeps pace with her growth and changing needs. Height, weight, and blood pressure should be taken at every one of those medical visits. A glycosylated hemoglobin test also should be done at those quarterly visits to help you and the doctor see the big picture of diabetes control. You should have access to diabetes educators—at least a nurse and a dietitian, and a mental health or counseling professional, if possible—who are experienced working with kids. See them regularly so that your diabetes management skills stay current and your child gets help learning to take control for herself in age-appropriate steps. Tests of blood lipids, kidney function, and the eyes should be done each year. This helps establish a baseline for comparison as your child gets older. It also helps make sure that any changes related to the diabetes are found very early, when treatment is generally simple and effective.

Build a good relationship with your child's diabetes health-care team. Obviously, your child's health-care team is extremely important to your success and comfort in dealing with diabetes. Different families want different types of relationships with their teams. Some need a lot of guidance— when a child is newly diagnosed or is going through a particularly difficult time, for example. Others prefer to be quite independent, with their team acting more as advisors. Your doctor and educators have important knowledge and skills to share with you. A good relationship allows you to benefit fully from that knowledge. On the other hand, if you have communication problems with the team or big differences in values about diabetes management, they won't be able to fill your needs. Because food is such a powerful and important area, make sure your team includes a dietitian who really knows both kids and diabetes. If it doesn't, ask your doctor for a referral.

There's quite a bit you can do to make sure you get what you need from your team. For example, be prepared when you go to appointments. Write down questions or problems you're having so you don't forget to mention them. Listen to the answers. Write down or ask for a written copy of any important instructions or information you're told. Speak up when you don't understand. No doctor or educator can answer every question, but they should be willing to find out or to help you figure out the problem. Nor can they know exactly what it's like to live with your child's diabetes, but they should be accepting and compassionate. As mentioned in the previous section, every doctor treating a child with diabetes should be aware of appropriate standards of care and should provide the necessary services.

The right health-care team is a treasure beyond price.

• • • •

If you're not getting what you need, speak up. Talking through any difficulties you're having is the first step to solving them. How your doctor and team respond to your concerns and questions should tell you whether the relationship can work for you. Changing doctors shouldn't be taken lightly. And sometimes it's not really an option, for example, for families whose health coverage is obtained through a managed care plan. But if the relationship isn't working, talk to your doctor or your insurance company representative about your choices. The right health-care team is a treasure beyond price. They will open doors, give you confidence, and become de facto members of the family. Without the right team on your side, however, you're fighting a formidable foe with inadequate weapons. David did beat Goliath, but it would have been easier with an UZI!

Give yourself credit for trying; mistakes are a necessary part of learning. Keep in mind that managing diabetes is a complicated skill that takes a long time to learn and even longer to master. All learning requires us to try new things. And trying something new means that we will make mistakes. Think back to when your child was learning to walk or to when you learned to ride a bike. Falling down was an inescapable part of the process. In fact, it was the falls that provided the feedback that you and the baby used to develop the ability to balance. Any baby who quit trying to walk after the first few falls would spend the rest of her days observing life from the seated position. And anyone who sees a hair-raising blood sugar reading as a sign of failure, instead of as a clue in a detective story, is going to feel frustrated and beaten a good deal of the time.

Compared to managing diabetes, walking and riding a bike are pretty simple skills, but the skill development process is exactly the same. It's been said that you have to be willing to do something badly in order to learn to do it well. That certainly is true of diabetes care. And while you're learning, give yourself and your child credit for trying. Try to treat the boo-boos, fiascoes, and near disasters of diabetes care like you did the baby's falls. A pat on the back, a hug, or a cheer keep the learning process going.

One of us has a young patient whose mother got very upset by her first effort to try the new, more liberal approach to including sweets in the meal plan. A dietitian talking about the new guidelines at a public lecture described a study in which quite a lot of chocolate cake was substituted in the diets of people with diabetes without impairing blood sugar control one iota. This was great news for Laurie, because the thing her son Cody had missed most since his diabetes was diagnosed was the great milk-chocolate cake from a neighborhood bakery. Laurie bought one of the cakes on the way home, and Cody had a nice big piece after dinner. Either the dietitian at the lecture had left out some important part of the puzzle or Cody's overall situation wasn't conducive to an extra piece of cake that night, because the next morning his blood sugar was 312 mg/dl.

"I should have known it was too good to be true," she moaned. "Now I'll have to chuck out the cake and tell Cody it was a false alarm." With a little discussion, however, we were able to redefine the episode as a learning opportunity and help Laurie cut herself a little slack. That first experiment with sweets wasn't a failure because it had shown them what doesn't work for Cody. It was the first step in figuring out what does work. And Mom needed credit for going to the lecture to learn more about diabetes and for caring enough to try something that would give Cody so much enjoyment.

We think the story of Thomas Edison and the lightbulb is a great image for how we need to look at diabetes self-care experiments that don't work out so well. Edison conducted over 5,000 experiments without succeeding in developing a lightbulb that worked. One day, a reporter came to his lab and asked why he didn't give up; how could he stand to fail 5,000 times? Edison replied, "I haven't failed once; I'm 5,000 steps closer to the solution."

Don't accept delivery of any guilt from health-care workers, family, and friends. Have you ever been busted by the "diabetes police"? You know who we mean. You're right on the edge to start with, pondering some deep, dark mystery of diabetes management—like how in the world that vegetable soup could have sent little Johnny's blood sugar into the stratosphere. Along comes well-meaning Aunt Flo. "You know, you really shouldn't be giving Johnny that white bread, Lucille. He should be getting more fiber with his diabetes and all." And you'd never really thought of yourself as a violent person before.

Diabetes police (DPs) come in many varieties: perfectionistic (health-care) providers, nosy neighbors, gloating grandmas, frank friends, and so on. They mean well. Their knowledge base may be excellent ("You should have given at least three extra units of Regular for that Otis Spunkmeyer muffin. You know, they have 50 grams of carbohydrate each.") or awful ("I just couldn't give my child shots every day. I heard if you gave them chromium supplements, they wouldn't need those terrible shots.") Whether their comments are helpful, hurtful, or just plain stupid, what they say puts you in a one-down position. They assume you're doing something wrong or that you're ignorant of some crucial fact of diabetes lore. And when these comments come at times when you're already feeling uncertain or frustrated, they really can add to your stress load.

You need a strategy for dealing with this type of input. Some parents tell us they just run a little tape in their heads; "He means well, but he doesn't know what he's talking about. We're doing the right thing." Others make their deflecting comments out loud; "I appreciate your concern, Mom, but we've discussed this with Jason's doctor. These foods are fine for his diabetes." Some let their DPs know exactly how they feel about the comments; "I get a little defensive when you make comments like that, Dad. We all work hard to take care of Troy's diabetes. It would help me a lot if you would ask us what's going on when you're concerned, instead of trying to give us advice."

Perhaps the hardest DPs to deal with are the perfectionistic providers, who have impossible expectations. These misguided souls are all too happy to berate parents when life with diabetes is human, that is to say, not perfect. You might try asking them if they know how few people in the DCCT intensive treatment group achieved normal blood sugars. Even with the best of care and support, only about 20% ever achieved a normal glycohemoglobin during the whole 9 years. Those who kept it normal made up only about 5 percent of the group. Tell them also that you're working hard to get the best control possible. Add that you sometimes feel pressured and even overwhelmed (or whatever your actual feelings are) by their standards, and that feeling that way makes it very difficult for you and your child to do your best.

The comeback that best protects you and your child while avoiding World War III will be different, depending on the source and the content of the comment. But however you respond, don't take delivery of the guilt. You don't deserve it, and it's not helpful.

Build an effective support system for yourself and your child.
Just as diabetes is too much for your child to handle alone, it is also likely to be too much for your family to handle alone.

When this is the case, get help. Some people hesitate to ask for help because they feel it will be a burden or an imposition, but this is seldom the case. People who care about you and your child will be willing to do whatever they can to help. In fact, they are likely to feel flattered by your confidence in them and certainly will feel closer to you as a result of the shared task of keeping the family well.

There are many possible sources of the support you need. Friends and extended family members can lighten the load tremendously. For many families, they are the logical source of the loving and knowledgeable child care that will allow Mom and Dad some relatively worry-free, personal time away from the demands of diabetes.

Join or start a support group for parents of kids with diabetes. There's no better outlet that we know of. The American Diabetes Association or Juvenile Diabetes Foundation chapters in your area may provide such services, and some hospitals and other organizations do, as well. And don't forget the support to your mental health that comes from the enjoyment of favorite hobbies and activities. Make some time for whatever gives you joy and relaxation. You'll have more to give and a better attitude as a result. You also might consider turning to your minister or rabbi or others you trust for support, advice, a shoulder to cry on, or anything else you feel you need.

Diabetes is a big load. Don't hesitate to reach out to other people for help. Remind yourself that asking for support is not a sign of weakness. It's a sign that you know how to take care of your child and yourself. And, incidentally, giving support to others when you can—in the family or through parent support groups, for example—is part of what makes a support system work. The give and take keeps everyone feeling as if they're getting what they need and not feeling as if they're being taken advantage of. One of the most important functions of a support system for the parents of kids with diabetes is that it makes taking our next piece of advice possible.

Take regular breaks from the diabetes by yourself and as a couple (or with other friends and family if you're a single parent). We're not sure if Mother Teresa ever takes a break from her labors. But living saints are in rather short supply. Most people who work at any emotion-laden task like dealing with a child's diabetes day in, day out must have a break now and again to maintain their own health and happiness. We've found that for many families, it takes at least a year after the diagnosis to start living more normally again. Exactly what's normal is unique to your own family, of course. Parents who were very active and had a booming social life B.D. (before diabetes), need to find a way to get back in the swing of things. On the other hand, moms and dads whose idea of a big night is renting a G-rated movie and munching popcorn with the kids, nestled in a big comforter in the middle of the living room floor, won't have as much of a change.

Take time to do things for your own health that you want your child to do for hers.

● ● ● ●

Some parents have a very hard time leaving their child with diabetes with another caregiver. They are too afraid something will go wrong in their absence. It seems that the younger the child is at diagnosis, the more difficult this is. If you are having this problem, it's important to find a way to overcome it, both for your good and for your child's. If you don't, you'll end up frazzled, and your fear and uncertainty may come across to your child. Train the baby-sitter or grandma. Make the first outings short and close to home to build your confidence. And, if necessary, get a beeper or cellular phone so you can be reached in an emergency. Do whatever it takes to get some time for yourself and for your relationship, free of the worries and demands of diabetes.

To repeat an important point we made before, your child with diabetes needs you happy and healthy. If you crash and burn, her most important teacher, advocate, and support is gone. If you won't take time for yourself for your own needs, do it for your child.

Protect your own physical health through good eating, enjoyable activity, and frequent laughter. Your body needs reasonable care and concern, too. Take time to do things for your own health that you want your child to do for hers. Managing diabetes is no job for weaklings. You need your strength—physical as well as mental—to cope. Eating well, as described in Chapter 3, is one important part of a healthy lifestyle that will keep you feeling your best. Getting a reasonable amount of physical activity is another. The variety of types and intensities of physical activity that different people would describe as the normal routine is extremely large. We've worked with families who would experience a 100% increase in physical activity if the battery in the TV remote control failed. And we've worked with families who consider 8 hours of scaling sheer cliffs with their bare hands a light family outing. They saved the really intense workouts for vacations trekking through Nepal or wilderness kayaking in Costa Rica. The very low level of activity described first is not likely to keep family members in good shape, and the very active lifestyle described second is much more exercise than anyone needs to stay optimally healthy. Personal preference, personality, access, and fitness level all affect the type and amount of activity that will be best for you.

But light aerobic activity—walking, jogging, bike riding, gardening, dancing, baseball, doubles tennis, roller blading, and so on—keeps the heart healthy, improves circulation, increases strength and endurance, and reduces tension. Try it. You'll like it! Kids raised in a physically active family are more likely to follow through with this as they grow.

And while you're out there jogging around the block and eating your cruciferous vegetables, have a good laugh now and then. It tones up muscles, lowers the blood pressure, improves the immune response, and makes you feel wonderful.

THE BOTTOM LINE

1. To help your child grow up healthy in every way, you must stay on an even keel yourself. Otherwise, the demands of diabetes on top of normal daily stresses may overwhelm you.

2. To maintain your own health and sanity, involve the whole family (and close friends) in living with diabetes. Give everyone a chance to help out.

3. Make sure your blood sugar goals for your child are realistic; trying to be perfect is a recipe for disaster.

4. Build a strong relationship with your child's diabetes health providers, and be sure she is getting the care she needs and deserves.

5. Take care of yourself; eat well, spend time with people you love, do things you enjoy, and laugh as often as possible.

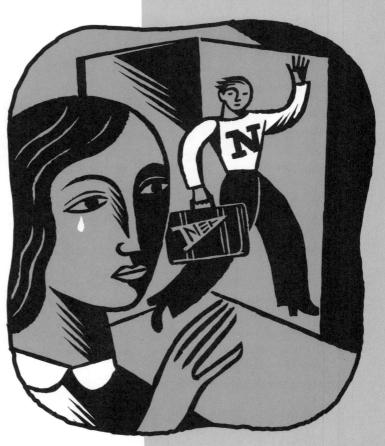

"Who's going to keep Russ out of DKA
now that he's going away to college?"

How to Help Your Child Learn to Control His Blood Sugars[1]

Both Russ and his mother were convinced that Mom was the only thing standing between the young man and utter disaster.

Russ was 20 when the time came for him to leave for college in Southern California. The inevitable had been delayed by a 2-year stay in the local junior college. Eventually, though, his ambition to be an architect required enrolling in a good design school that was some 400 miles from home. As the day of departure came closer, he and his mother became more and more frantic.

Both Russ and his mother were convinced that Mom was the only thing standing between the young man and utter disaster. Unlike most of the teenagers we see, Russ hadn't tried very hard to break away from Mom's control of his diabetes during his adolescence. With brief and minor exceptions, he had kept a very regular schedule for a teenager, carefully

---

[1] Based on Rubin RR: Working with diabetic adolescents. In *Practical Psychology for Diabetes Clinicians.* Anderson BJ, Rubin RR, Eds. Alexandria, VA, American Diabetes Association, 1996.

279

counted his grams of carbohydrate to fulfill the meal plan, tested fairly often, and reviewed the numbers with his Mom when blood sugars got too out of whack. A "perfect" (and unusual!) child.

Mom was an extremely accomplished diabetes caregiver. Her skillful adjustments of insulin and activity had kept Russ's diabetes on an even keel for years. She managed the diabetes during illness better than the vast majority of endocrine resident physicians. She and Russ felt very safe with the setup and were equally fearful that their coming separation would spell real trouble.

You might say that Mrs. Lear had become the world's expert on her child's diabetes. This is a commendable accomplishment. But, unfortunately, she had stopped short of fulfilling her complete task. She had neglected, out of love and worry, to help Russ learn to control his own blood sugars. So, at age 20, Russ was getting the very short course in diabetes self-management. The skills themselves were not hard to teach him. But without a lot of time to practice those skills in a safe environment, Russ was going off to college with an unnecessary load of worry and risk. And Mom was having the devil's own time letting go. The only thing that was keeping her from moving to Los Angeles ("Just for the first semester or two until I'm sure he's okay.") was her husband's angry insistence that he wasn't about to pay for two apartments in L.A.

As you know so well, diabetes cannot be controlled by health-care providers. Diabetes is controlled at home, at the soccer game, at school...not in the doctor's office or hospital. The people who are there have to have the skill. If you break your arm or develop a bad infection, your recovery depends almost entirely on the doctor's skill in choosing and applying the right therapy. Did he set the arm correctly? Did he pick the right antibiotic to attack the infection? But in diabetes, the success of therapy depends much less on the skill of the doctor in picking the therapy than it does on the ability of the child and the family to put the therapy to work in the real world.

Mrs. Lear understood this. But she hadn't been able to pass on her own expertise to the most important person in this equation: Russ.

You wouldn't want someone who didn't know what he was doing to set your broken arm or take out your inflamed appendix. And likewise, you don't want the person taking care of your child's diabetes to be incapable and unsure. You want someone competent and confident to make those daily management decisions. But as we've pointed out before, you can't be that person as your child grows up and goes away. That would not be good for you or for your child. For your child to grow and develop normally into an independent adult, that capable and confident diabetes manager has to be the child himself. Building the needed skill requires taking small steps from a very young age and progressively larger ones as the years go by until the child has all the skills necessary for his own safety and well-being.

If you keep in mind the fact that your job is to help your child learn to control his blood sugars and not to control them yourself, you'll appreciate the benefits of helping him learn what works for his diabetes and his life. He probably wants to be as free of his diabetes as possible, and that's understandable. He wants to do the things other kids do. He wants to enjoy birthday parties, sleep over at friends' houses, and be as unencumbered by his diabetes as he can be. These are normal and achievable goals, and you can help him reach them. Doing your part means sympathizing with him when he's upset, helping him solve problems when he's stuck, praising him as often as possible, criticizing him as infrequently as possible, and loving him all the time.

Helping your child learn self-control requires being clear about the difference between pushing and supporting. Everyone likes support, but no one likes to be pushed. When you support your child, you are helping him reach a goal he has chosen; when you push him, you are trying to get him to do something you have chosen. And when you push, as we pointed out earlier, your child is very likely to resist. We aren't suggesting that you let your child make diabetes management decisions on his own, but we are suggesting that you let him take the lead in making these decisions. You are there to keep him out of trouble as he does this, to be sure, but you are giving him the chance to safely practice the life-giving skills he will need in the years to come.

This approach can be hard for parents. They fear their child will not do the right thing when it comes to diabetes care. And he might not, all of the time. But he'll do fine most of the time, if you work together with love and mutual respect, gradually shifting responsibility to him. Never forget, if your child doesn't buy into the diabetes care plan you think he should, he somehow will find a way to use his veto power anyway. Helping him learn to make his own decisions is really the only way to go.

In the meantime, you might keep in mind the words of the Serenity Prayer: "God grant me the serenity to accept the things I cannot change, the courage to change the things I can, and the wisdom to know the difference." When you live by this credo, you are doing everything within your power to help your child live a happy, healthy life, and you keep the love flowing between you as well.

Your child and his diabetes are unique. There are no cookbooks for diabetes management or for your child's development. You have to develop your own recipe. This means first learning the theory and techniques through reading books, taking classes, working with a diabetes educator, going to support groups, and so on. Then, using the techniques in this chapter, engage your child in his care while passing on your skill and confidence in a safe environment. We call this process facilitating self-control.

PARENTING TECHNIQUES THAT FACILITATE SELF-CONTROL IN DIABETES

Ask questions. Questions are the most powerful tool you have for helping your child grow up healthy and happy. They're also terrific for preserving the peace in the meantime. We introduce you to this idea in Chapter 5, when we talk about how Sally and her mother solved the Christmas cookie problem. Asking questions is the foundation for your parent-child diabetes care partnership, an essential strategy for passing on skill and responsibility to your child in a safe way.

Some of the questions you need to ask are unique to your family, while others are common to many families who live with diabetes. Among the latter are questions such as, "What's the hardest thing for you right now about managing your diabetes?," "Is there anything I can do to help?," and "What do you think we should do about this problem?" What all these questions have in common is that they are open-ended invitations to your child to share his thoughts.

When it comes to good questions, tone and timing are crucial. We're reminded of a 12-year-old named Tiffany, whose mother was beside herself because her daughter would never (according to Mom) test her blood before dinner without a major hassle. Mom said she'd tried everything: getting the testing supplies and sitting with Tiffany trying to force her to do the test, refusing to give her daughter dinner until she had done the test, and punishing her for not doing the test; all to no avail. Tiffany agreed that the situation was awful.

When the nurse asked Tiffany if she thought testing her blood before dinner was important, Tiffany said yes. She was at a loss, though, to explain exactly why she didn't test. Part of it was that she didn't like interrupting what she was doing to test. Part of it was that she hated having her mother tell her what to do. All the same, she acknowledged that she would probably not test on her own. It seemed there was no way out. Still, the nurse asked Tiffany if she could think of any way for her mother to help her test. After a little thought, Tiffany suggested an experiment: if her mother would ask her 10 minutes before dinner if she had tested, she would try to follow through.

When Tiffany and her mom came to their next clinic appointment, Tiffany's mother blurted out, "Well, that idea certainly didn't work!" She went on to say that she had forgotten to ask Tiffany about her test for the first few days after their last visit. She finally remembered on the 4th day, but only after dinner had already begun. At this point, she turned to Tiffany and said, "You didn't test, did you?!" Tone and timing. Tone and timing. Tiffany's mom missed on both counts. Instead of being a supportive reminder, the question came out as an aggressive put-down.

She had asked what we sometimes call a rhetorical question, one to which she already knew (or thought she knew) the answer. Another example of a rhetorical question might be, "Did you eat those cookies that were on the counter?" when your child has high blood sugar and chocolate crumbs on her T-shirt.

When you ask questions, make them real ones. Ask questions designed to open up communication with your child, to give you information, and to help him take better care of himself. Avoid questions designed to blame or to catch your child making mistakes of judgment or behavior.

Learn from successes. There will be times when a problem situation goes more smoothly than usual. One of the most important and useful questions you can ask at times like this is "How come that worked so well?" Figuring out exactly what helped can be tremendously beneficial. Let's say your child usually finds it hard to limit himself to the amount he's supposed to eat for his afternoon snack. Then one day he's fine with what you give him. Understanding what made this day different from all others provides both of you with invaluable information. Maybe your child was involved with something he really enjoyed doing, maybe he was less hungry than usual, or maybe he just ate his snack earlier than normal. The specific factor will be different for different kids. Puzzling out what made things go well will help your child learn effective strategies for controlling his diabetes. And it will help him learn in the best possible way, by focusing on his successes rather than his failures.

Individualize. We can't repeat too often the fact that the best plan for managing diabetes in your family must take into account the unique individuals involved. Some kids really like routines, while others hate them. Some children have few problems eating what's provided in the amounts offered, others can't live with the limits their meal plans impose, and still others are such picky eaters that their parents live in constant dread of hypoglycemia. Some kids are totally at ease managing their diabetes in public, eating their snacks, taking their shots, and doing their tests no matter who notices. Others want as few people as possible to know about their diabetes, and they wouldn't dream of taking a shot or doing a blood test in front of anyone. Some children feel their diabetes is an almost overwhelming burden, and others say it's more like a moderate inconvenience. And the aspect of having diabetes that's most bothersome varies, as well. For one child it might be shots, for another, doctor's appointments or blood tests, not being able to eat as much candy as his friends, or having to stop during ball games for a snack. The list of potential individual differences is endless. The point is, the only problems you and your child need to solve are the ones you actually have. Try to identify and work on the diabetes-related issues that cause the most stress in your family.

Individualize your goals as well. If you like, you can refer to Chapter 5, where we talk about picking "good enough" blood sugar goals for your child and family. When you are working toward those goals, keep in mind that some kids simply have an easier time getting good blood sugars than other kids do. This is especially true of those who are recently diagnosed. They are likely to still be in what we call the "honeymoon" phase of their diabetes, when the pancreas is still producing some insulin. That small amount of body insulin makes blood sugars much more stable and easier to control than they will be later on, when the last of the body's insulin disappears.

Another type of child who has a relatively easier time of controlling blood sugars is the one who tends to be unusually regular in his daily pattern of eating, exercise, insulin administration, and sleeping. And there are other kids whose relative ease in achieving good blood sugar control can't be explained. Whatever the reason, if your child seems to get good blood sugar numbers without much effort, your individual goals can be a bit more ambitious than if his diabetes were more difficult to manage.

Unfortunately, most kids don't have such an easy time of it. If your child is a teenager, if he is less given to routines, if he has trouble easily achieving good blood sugar control for any reason, you must adjust your goals accordingly. These goals should still be ambitious, to be sure, but they must also be realistic. Otherwise, you and your child will end up miserable and discouraged. And this discouragement will actually make the best control he can manage even harder to achieve.

Be specific. As you work with your child toward your common goals, the more detail you identify as you define problems, vulnerabilities, strengths, and successes, the easier life will be. Here's a story that makes the point. Rita was a high school senior. She had been diagnosed with diabetes at the age of 7 and had managed it well. Suddenly, she started running really high blood sugars. In fact, she was so hyperglycemic many mornings that she couldn't even drag herself out of bed to go to school. It turned out that Rita was going to the mall every night after dinner and hanging out with her friends. One of their favorite activities, other than talking, was eating. Rita joined in, and by the time she got home, her blood sugar was sky high. For some reason, at this point, Rita told herself that it was "too late" to do anything about the hyperglycemia and just went to bed. As a result, she was up half the night urinating, and she was in big trouble the next morning. The fact that Rita could acknowledge she had a problem and that she could be so specific in describing it was very helpful in finding a solution.

Naturally, the solution had to be equally specific, and Rita was very clear about some potential solutions that would not work for her: She *would not* 1) stop going to the mall, 2) stop eating when she went to the mall, 3) carry all her insulin paraphernalia with her to the mall, and 4) take an extra shot when she got home. Though in a way Rita was being difficult, in another way she was being helpful. She was making it crystal clear what would not work. The physician to whom Rita described her problem appreciated Rita's openness, and he racked his brain to come up with a solution. After offering a few suggestions that Rita vetoed, he came up with one she was willing to try: carry an insulin pen containing Regular insulin to the mall in her purse. Rita said she would go to the bathroom right before she ate and give herself from one to four units to cover the food she had ordered. This worked for her because she could do it so quickly.

When you work toward specific solutions with your child, keep this image in mind: If you can help your child describe a problem (or a solution) so specifically that you could make a movie of it, you are on the right track. Getting that specific often takes time and work. It involves asking deeper and deeper questions about a situation, trying to discover what's really going on as you might seek to solve a mystery. Approaching a problem in this spirit is often very effective. Think about the energy your child is willing to invest in things that really interest him (like how to get the girl he has a crush on to notice him, for example). Wouldn't it be wonderful if he could tap that same energy and curiosity in his efforts to learn to manage his diabetes?

Another benefit of defining problems as specifically as possible is that it makes living with diabetes feel more manageable. Many people are relieved when they are able to see clearly that their sticking point is some specific, manageable piece of the diabetes regimen rather than the whole thing.

Take a step-by-step approach. Any problem is easier to solve when you break it down into manageable steps. Diabetes-related problems are no exception. Think of any situation that you want to work on: helping your child begin doing his own shots, for example. Then think of all the steps involved in actually completing that task: getting out the insulin, choosing a syringe, deciding how much insulin to give (if you are using a sliding scale), cleaning the top of the vial, drawing up the insulin, checking to make sure you have drawn up the right amount, giving the shot, writing down the amount of insulin you have given, and, finally, putting everything back where it belongs.

Once you've made the list of steps, tell your child he can pick any one step he wants to do himself. (Naturally you want to make sure he picks one that he can actually handle, or one that you can closely monitor). Once he is comfortable taking responsibility for the first task he chose (this may take a couple of days or a couple of weeks), ask him which step he wants to assume next. In this way, you help him learn the skills he needs to master one step at a time, with you there to make sure he is doing things right. This allows you to shift diabetes care responsibility to your child step-by-step, so it's easy for him to manage. Almost any diabetes regimen responsibility can be broken down into steps and transferred this way.

This gentle, gradual approach to helping your child learn to manage his own diabetes also lets you stay in touch with an older child, increasing the likelihood that nothing important will slip between the cracks. Stefan, whom you met in the **Introduction: When It's Your Child With Diabetes**, has been using an insulin pump since he was 11 years old. When he was 20, just before he moved out on his own, his dad was still helping when it was time to change the insulin pump infusion set and refill the pump syringe. Stefan didn't really need the help, but it was a wonderful opportunity to check on how things were going diabetes-wise. It was also a chance for Stefan and his dad to remind themselves that diabetes management was something they would always share. From the youngest child to the oldest, taking a step-by-step approach to shifting responsibility for diabetes care is the way to go. It builds confidence (in both parent and child), facilitates independence, ensures that diabetes management tasks are all attended to, and strengthens your relationship, all at the same time.

Here's one more tip for making the step-by-step approach work for your family. As you begin to divide up responsibilities for a task, don't just check up on your child; have him check up on you, too. Let him verify that you have drawn up the right amount of insulin, chosen the proper foods for his lunch, or taken everything you will need for your trip to the park. That way you convey the cooperative nature of diabetes care, and you help your child begin to learn what he needs to know with a minimum of pressure.

Do regular reality and comfort checks. Keeping on top of diabetes takes maintenance, so it's important to check in regularly with your child to see how he feels things are going. Ask him about any new problems that might have come up, about any successes he's had managing his diabetes, and about anything you might have noticed that you feel needs discussion. Some families find it works well to have a regular diabetes family meeting where everyone gets to say anything they want about how things have been going since the last meeting. This can be a good opportunity to deal with small problems before they become big ones. The key to success with these meetings is maintaining an attitude of cooperation.

Maintaining contact is especially important as your child gets older and assumes more of the day-to-day management of his diabetes. Remember what we said about how some aspects of the regimen can go undone if you give them up before your child is fully prepared to take them on. Regular contact and continued involvement can help avoid trouble.

You will also want to maintain contact with other adults who regularly have responsibility for your child. This might include teachers, coaches, youth group leaders, and others. Naturally, you want your child to know when you speak to these folks. He might even want to be with you when you do. As we discussed earlier, these adults need to be well-versed in managing potential diabetes-related emergencies, of which hypoglycemia is the most obvious example. Once you've provided the information, it's important to check in occasionally to see if any problems have come up that you need to know about. We cover some of the specifics of ensuring your child is well cared for at school in Chapter 11.

Support problem-solving skills. We want our children to know they can do anything they set their minds to, as long as they are willing to solve the problem of how to do it safely. Stefan, the young man we talked about earlier, personifies effective diabetes problem-solving. At the age of 11, just a few days after he got his insulin pump, his dad took him to visit a friend in New York City. The friend never cooked meals at home, so dinner at a local restaurant was planned. Stefan talked his father into letting him order anything he wanted on the menu—it was, after all, a special occasion—but when Stefan tested his blood just before ordering, his meter read 350 mg/dl. Stefan's dad knew the boy wanted to order coconut custard pie with ice cream for dessert, and the nervous parent's mind was swimming with images of a midnight visit to a local emergency room. We all would have understood it if Dad had followed his first instinct to go back on his agreement. But he didn't.

Instead, he decided to take a chance on his son's budding diabetes problem-solving skills, and maybe even strengthen them in the process. Dad said he would stick with the agreement on the condition that Stefan think really hard about how much insulin he needed to take, and that he test his blood 2 hours and 4 hours after dinner.

Stefan readily agreed and then proceeded to eat a big dinner complete with that slice of coconut custard pie à la mode. At 2 hours later, his blood sugar was 220 mg/dl, and at 4 hours later, it was 170 mg/dl. Stefan and his dad were both delighted with the outcome, of course. His dad asked Stefan how he had managed to figure out the amount of insulin he needed to cover the meal. The boy explained that he'd used the formula he'd been taught to calculate the insulin dose based on the amount of carbohydrate eaten. "I really wanted that food, Dad, and I certainly didn't want to feel sick later, so I was very careful when I counted the food. Working hard, like that, is worth it when I can see I got the insulin right."

You can support problem-solving by asking your child questions. How can you (or he) safely do that thing you've got your heart set on? Even if something goes wrong, remember to give credit for the effort. Then ask questions to learn as much as possible from the experience. You'll have a better starting point the next time a similar situation arises. And if something went right, try to find out why so you can learn from that experience, too.

Build emotional strength. Dealing effectively with diabetes requires emotional strength, as well as problem-solving skills. We've found that the fundamental elements of this emotional strength are love, faith, and humor. If you can foster these qualities in yourself, and nurture them in your child, you will do well in your lives with diabetes.

It is said that love conquers all, and when it comes to coping with the stress of life with diabetes, this may well be true. Love gives us confidence, and it just plain feels wonderful. Best of all, the more love you give, the more you get. Make sure the hassles and aggravations of daily life with diabetes don't prevent you from enjoying, appreciating, and loving your child as fully as you can. A 9-year-old we know went through a period when he decided that his shots would hurt less if he did them slowly. Now, when we say slowly, we mean very, very, very slowly. Often, his mother would sit with him in the morning for 5 minutes or more as he pressed the needle to his skin. The need to get him moving toward school made this performance even harder for her to bear. She wisely kept her frustration to herself, but one day she reached her limit.

She said, "I know those shots must really hurt. Even just watching you, I get a knot in my stomach. I love you so much, if I could take half your shots for you, I would." Her son looked at her quizzically for a moment. Then he responded, "It doesn't hurt that much, Mom," and he pushed the needle right in. Turns out he had hit a rough spot, and he was temporarily stuck. But all he needed was that little boost that came from knowing he was loved. In fact, he never went back to his slow-motion injection method.

Faith is another bulwark against the stresses and strains of daily life with diabetes. If you and your child have faith in a higher power, you can draw on the strength it provides you. There's also the faith you can foster in modern medical technology, in your diabetes health-care providers, and, most importantly, in yourselves. A woman we know was diagnosed with diabetes over 40 years ago. No one in her family had ever had diabetes before, so it was unknown territory for all of them. When the girl asked her mother what having diabetes would mean for them, her mom responded, "It means we will learn to eat better than we have ever eaten before, and we will all be healthier than we ever were before, and we will all learn to love each other more than we ever did before." Now that's faith.

Another boy, who was 11 years old, was sitting with his father talking about things they wished for. When his father said he wished his son didn't have diabetes, the boy said, "I don't wish that. Not that I like diabetes; in fact, I hate it. But having diabetes has forced me to learn how to take care of myself. I can take care of myself better than any of my friends, and I wouldn't give that up for anything in the world."

For a few days, before you go to sleep each night, remind yourself of three things you did that day to help your child live a better life with diabetes.

● ● ● ●

When we succeed in helping our children have faith in themselves, we are giving them one of life's most precious gifts. It will help them live well with their diabetes and with all the other challenges they will face in life. Naturally, to help your child have faith, you must have it yourself. Think of the things that buoy you up. Think of the things from which you draw strength and inspiration. If you have trouble doing this, try the following exercise.

For a few days, before you go to sleep each night, remind yourself of three things you did that day to help your child live a better life with diabetes. Then remind yourself of three things your child did to work toward the same goal. All too often, we lose sight of our accomplishments and successes. Bringing them to mind can help keep us strong and build our confidence.

Humor is wonderful. Along with faith and love, it's the closest thing to magic in the world. How often have you heard someone say, "I don't know how I would have made it if it hadn't been for my sense of humor"? You may have even said it yourself. Humor helps you keep things in perspective; it protects you from feeling overwhelmed. If you can help your child apply humor to his life with diabetes, it will give him a boost. A 10-year-old we know was really upset when he had to start taking an extra insulin shot each day. When he was first diagnosed, he was taking just one shot each morning, but soon his physician recommended adding a second shot at dinnertime. Unfortunately, the boy did not take well to the second shot. In fact, he pitched a fit every night, wondering quite loudly why he couldn't go on taking just one shot a day. For several weeks his mother kept answering the question. She explained, over and over and in ever-increasing detail, the benefits of that second shot. All to no avail. Finally, one night she decided a new approach was called for.

When her son asked his nightly question, "Why can't I take just one shot a day?" she responded, "I can't think of any reason. But why stop with one shot a day, how about one shot a week?" Getting into the swing of things, her son suggested one shot a month, and his mother came back, "Let's go for the whole ball of wax: one shot a year."

Laughing, the boy retorted, "But think about how big the syringe would have to be!" The youngster, who was good in math, quickly calculated the answer: 12,775 units. One heck of a syringe! The boy took that evening shot without a fuss, and he did the same the next evening and every evening after that. Apparently, the evening shot was not the real problem; the shot was simply the straw that broke the camel's back. It marked the point at which the boy went from barely managing to being frankly overwhelmed. Like any human being, he looked up and saw the final straw of the load that had flattened him and said, "That's my problem." But it really wasn't; being overwhelmed was the problem, not the second shot. What the boy was really saying was not, "Why do I have to take a second shot?" He was really saying, "I'm overwhelmed. Help me lighten the load." Humor can do that, and it did.

Sometimes, your child herself may be the source of the humor. A 7-year-old girl was on a camping trip with her parents in a very beautiful and very isolated area.

Unfortunately, on the 2nd day of their vacation, a huge storm struck, drenching their tent and soaking through to reach them and all of their equipment. To make matters worse, at the height of the storm the girl had a terrible episode of low blood sugar. Her blood sugar was so low that she could not swallow anything, and her parents had to give her a shot of glucagon, which they had been wise enough to pack. This brought their daughter to consciousness, but as they tried to feed her to keep her blood sugar up, she began to vomit. And she vomited, and she vomited, and she vomited. For hours she sat there soaking wet with her head in a bucket. Her parents, equally wet, were rapidly losing their minds. Finally, the girl leaned over the bucket yet again, and her father felt as if he was on the verge of losing it altogether. At that very moment, his daughter lifted her head, smiled wanly, and said, "Oh, bad day." At this her parents started to laugh. After a moment, their daughter joined in, and soon they were all feeling much, much better.

Remember your goal: a happy, healthy, independent child who will love you forever.

● ● ● ●

The essence of humor is taking a bad situation and exaggerating its awfulness to the point where it's so ridiculous it becomes funny. Fortunately or unfortunately, life with diabetes presents us with plenty of material for humor. Try to find some in your daily life and see what you can make of it.

Remember your goal: a happy, healthy, independent child who will love you forever (even when you are 90 and he is 65). When you continue to love him and support him and stay involved with his diabetes as he grows to young adulthood, you are increasing your chances of reaching your goal. You are helping your child learn to be strong, confident, and open. Managing food and nutrition is just a part of that overall picture of a well-functioning family. When you do your part of the job—getting the right food on the table and, in a more general way, helping him learn to control his own blood sugars—you have accomplished a very great deal. He will then be able to manage what he can manage on his own and ask for your help when he needs it. What more can we ask?

THE BOTTOM LINE

1. Your job is to help your child learn to control his own diabetes. Kids are never too young to begin taking part in their own care, and they are never too old to benefit from some support from their parents. Start working cooperatively when your child is young, and stay involved through his teen years.
2. Asking good questions is the most powerful tool you have for helping your child learn to control his own blood sugars.
3. Everyone learns best from successes, so focus on what your child does right rather than what he does wrong.
4. Your child is unique. Make sure you work to help your child develop specific, step-by-step approaches to the problems that bother him most.
5. Emotional strength, based on love, faith, and humor, is fundamental for living well with diabetes. Foster these qualities in yourself, and nurture them in your child.

Index

G

Glucagon injections, 149–150, 154, 214
Glucose, 64–65
    tablets/gel, 148
Glycosylated hemoglobin, 91–92, 94–97
    testing yearly, 269
Grains, 48–50
Great Depression, 16–17
Growth
    blood glucose control and, 38–39, 93–94, 242–243
    food intake measurement and, 31–37
    genetic potential for, 34–36, 256
    height/weight relationship, 36
    of infants, 208–211
    questions for health-care team, 37
    of teenagers, 242–243
    of toddlers, 218
Growth grids
    for children, 32–36
    for infants, 208–210
Growth hormones, 97, 242

H

HbA$_{1c}$. *See* Glycosylated hemoglobin
Health-care team
    infants and, 207
    minimum medical visits/tests, 268–269
    pregnancy needs and, 256
    relationship with, 269–270
    teenagers and, 244, 256
    unrealistic expectations of, 273
Healthy eating, 13–23. *See also* Nutrition
    barriers to, 186–187
    changing to, 44–45, 199
    child's role in, 21–22, 196, 197–198
    environmental control for, 199
    expectations and, 200
    parents' role in, 15–16, 19–21, 195–198, 258–259

for whole family, 20–21, 43–44, 198–199
Heart, exercise and, 159
Height, weight and, 36
Herskowitz-Dumont, Raymonde, 161
Honeymoon period, 160, 285
Hormones, counterregulatory, 131–132, 134–135, 149
    adrenaline, 132, 163, 254
    cortisol, 132
    defined, 131
    glucagon, 132, 149
    growth, 97, 242
    stress, 97
Humalog insulin, 139–140, 142
Humor, 183, 276, 292–294
Hyperglycemia, 93
    exercise and, 162–163
    prevention of, 115
    snacks and, 122–124
Hypoglycemia, 93, 129–155
    causes of
        activity, 143
        alcohol consumption, 143–144, 251–252
        excessive insulin, 137–139
        food, too little, 139–143
        intensive diabetes treatment, 98–99, 136–137
        menstrual cycle, 144
        sexual activity, 254–255
    defined, 131
    driving and, 252
    exercise-induced, 162
        recognition/prevention, 171–172
        in very young children, 173–174
    glucagon injections, 149–150, 154, 214
    in infants, 212–214
    intensive diabetes treatment and, 98–99, 136–137
    levels of, 133–134
    mild, 133, 146–147
    moderate, 133, 147–149
    nighttime, 152–153
    prevention of
        blood glucose goal adjustment, 136–137

N

O

T

Taste preferences, 41–43, 54–57, 196
Teenagers, 241–259
  alcohol consumption by, 250–252
  appetite of, 248–250
  blood glucose control and, 96–97, 242–243
    motivation for, 256–257
  calorie needs of, 248–250
  challenges, 241–243
  contraception, 254–255
  doctor visits, 244
  driving risks, 252
  drugs and, 253–254
  eating habits, criticism of, 243–244
  emotional changes in, 243–244
  family meals and, 258–259
  growth of, 242–243, 256
  insulin pumps for, 247, 257–258
  insulin requirements, 242–243
  intensive diabetes treatment for, 257
  late nights, 246–247
  peer relationships, 245–246
  portion sizes for, 49
  pregnancy, 255–256
  privacy for, 244
  schedule problems, 246–248
  self-care by, 108, 243
  sex and, 254–256
  sleeping late, 247–248
  tobacco use, 252–253
Time block method, of meal planning, 116–118, 232–233
Tobacco, 252–253
Toddlers, 216–221
  artificially sweetened drinks and, 219
  blood glucose monitoring, 220
  characteristics of, 216–217
  exercise and, 172–174
  feeding of, 217–219
    force-feeding, 217
    portion sizes for, 49
    setting limits, 218
    snacks, 219
    sweets, 219

  vegetarian diets, 52
  insulin management, 220
Total available glucose (TAG), 68
Type I diabetes
  and alcohol consumption, 251
  DCCT participants, 94–95
  exercise benefits and, 160

U

Ultralente insulin
  absorption variability, 137–138
  adjustments for exercise, 168–169
  food acceptance problems and, 141
  nighttime hypoglycemia and, 120, 152–153
  sleeping late and, 248
Unawareness, hypoglycemia, 135
Urine testing
  for glucose, 211–212
  for ketones, 163–164, 212

V

Vegetables, 48, 50
  portion sizes by age, 49
Vegetarian diets, 51–53
Vitamin B12, vegetarian diets and, 52
Vitamin supplements, vegetarian diets and, 52

W

Wallet cards, medical alert, 150–151
Weight control. *See also* Clinical eating disorders
  activity levels and, 27
  attitudes toward, 194
  exercise and, 160, 178
  intensive diabetes treatment and, 99–100
  obesity, 27, 160
  teenagers and, 250
  by withholding food, 17–18
Withholding food, 17–18

• • • •

The American Diabetes Association Library of Self-Care and Nutrition

SELF-CARE

American Diabetes Association Complete Guide to Diabetes

When you want information on diabetes self-care you usually have to turn to several books, each covering a different topic: nutrition, blood sugar, exercise, complications, etc. Finally, *all* areas of self-care are covered in the pages of *one* book. Complete, thorough chapters cover every aspect of self-care. You'll learn all about symptoms and causes ... diagnosis and treatment ... handling emergencies ... complications and prevention ... achieving good blood sugar control ... and more. You'll also discover advice on nutrition, exercise, sex, pregnancy, family life, travel, coping, and health insurance. #CSMCGD

Nonmember: $29.95; ADA Member: $23.95

Raising a Child With Diabetes

Having diabetes doesn't mean your child has to sit on the sidelines. Gone are the bland diets and poor excuses for missing gym class. You'll learn how to help your child adjust insulin to allow for foods kids like to eat, have a busy schedule and still feel healthy and strong, negotiate the twists and turns of being "different," accept the physical and emotional challenges life has to offer, and much more. Through periods of picky eating, sick days, and times when your child is reluctant to do a blood test or take an injection, you now have a helpful companion at your side, every step of the way. #CSMRCWD

Nonmember: $14.95; ADA Member: $11.95

The Dinosaur Tamer and Other Stories for Children With Diabetes

Danny Littleton feels like he is turning into a dinosaur every time he goes to the doctor's office. After all, dinosaurs don't have to be afraid of anything, including having diabetes. The doctor understands how Danny feels. He and Danny talk, and later, in school, Danny realizes that if he pretends he is a dinosaur, he can get up in front of the class and explain his diabetes. *The Dinosaur Tamer* is just one of 25 fictional stories that will entertain, enlighten, and ease your child's frustrations about having diabetes. Ages 8-12. #CSMDTAOS

Nonmember: $9.95; ADA Member: $7.95

COOKING AND NUTRITION

Diabetic Meals in 30 Minutes—Or Less!

Here are more than 140 quick-and-easy, good-for-you recipes you can put on the table in a hurry. In about 20 minutes you can sit down to the sumptuous aroma of South-of-the-Border Chicken. Or treat yourself to a little taste of Italy with Chicken Rigatoni. Put Oven-Baked Parmesan Zucchini on the table in 20 minutes. Then let it melt in your mouth. The 10-Minute Vinaigrette Dressing adds just the right tangy bite to salad greens. And the left-overs will keep in the refrigerator for two whole weeks! Still room for dessert? Throw Layered Vanilla Yogurt Parfait together in no time at all. Then take your sweet time enjoying it. So whether you're looking for quick-to-fix appetizers, desserts, soups, salads, or entrees, you'll find them all in *Diabetic Meals in 30 Minutes—Or Less!* #CCBDM

Nonmember: $11.95; ADA Member: $9.95

Diabetes Meal Planning Made Easy

Meal planning can often be the most difficult part of managing diabetes. But, the new Diabetes Food Pyramid makes meal planning easier than ever. And now you can discover the new diabetes nutrition recommendations and how to master the intricacies of each food group in the new Diabetes Food Pyramid. From starches, at the pyramid's base, to fats, sweets, and alcohol at the pyramid's tip, you'll learn how much of what foods to eat to fit your personal needs. You'll also learn how to skim fat and eat less meat; make realistic changes in your eating habits; use quick and easy ways to eat more starches, fruits, vegetables, and milk; incorporate strategies to fit preplanning into your schedule; accurately read the Nutrition Facts on food labels; use practical tips for eating away from home; much more. #CCBMP

Nonmember: $14.95; ADA Member: $11.95

The Healthy HomeStyle Cookbook

Here are more than 150 healthy recipes with old-fashioned great taste. Try Chicken Nuggets, Sweet and Sour Meatballs, Sloppy Joes, Dutch Apple Pancakes, Oven-Fried Onion Rings, Macaroni and Cheese, Crispy Baked Chicken, and more. Complete nutrition information accompanies every recipe. Special "lay-flat" binding allows hands-free reference while you cook. Alphabetized index helps you find your favorites in a snap. #CCBHS

Nonmember: $12.50; ADA Member: $9.95

Month of Meals

When celebrations begin, go ahead—dig in! The original "automatic menu planner" includes a Special Occasion section that offers tips for brunches, holidays, parties, and restaurants to give you delicious dining options anytime, anywhere. Menu choices include Chicken Cacciatore, Oven Fried Fish, Sloppy Joes, Crab Cakes, and many others. #CMPMOM

Nonmember: $12.50; ADA Member: $9.95

Month of Meals 2

Automatic menu planning goes ethnic! A healthy diet doesn't have to keep you from your favorite restaurants. Tips and meal suggestions for Mexican, Italian, and Chinese restaurants are featured. Quick-to-fix and ethnic recipes are also included. Menu choices include Beef Burritos, Chop Suey, Veal Piccata, Stuffed Peppers, and many others. #CMPMOM2

Nonmember: $12.50; ADA Member: $9.95

Month of Meals 3

Enjoy fast food without guilt! Make sensible but delicious choices at McDonald's, Wendy's, Taco Bell, Kentucky Fried Chicken, and other fast-food restaurants. Special sections offer valuable tips, such as reading ingredient labels, preparing meals for picnics, and meal planning when you're ill. Menu choices include Fajita in a Pita, Seafood Stir Fry, Stouffer's Macaroni and Cheese, and many others. #CMPMOM3

Nonmember: $12.50; ADA Member: $9.95

Month of Meals 4

Meat and potatoes menu planning! Beef up your meal planning with old-time family favorites like Meatloaf and Pot Roast, Crispy Fried Chicken, Beef Stroganoff, Kielbasa and Sauerkraut, Sausage and Cornbread Pie, and many others. Hints for turning family-size meals into delicious left-overs will keep generous portions from going to waste. Meal plans for one or two people are also featured. Spiral-bound. #CMPMOM4

Nonmember: $12.50; ADA Member: $9.95

Month of Meals 5

Meatless meals picked fresh from the garden! Choose from a garden of fresh vegetarian selections like Eggplant Italian, Stuffed Zucchini, Cucumbers with Dill Dressing, Vegetable

Lasagna, and many others. Plus, you'll reap all the health benefits of a vegetarian diet, including less obesity, less coronary artery disease, less colon and lung cancer, less osteoporosis, and more. #CMPMOM5

Nonmember: $12.50; ADA Member: $9.95

Great Starts & Fine Finishes

Begin dinner with Crab-Filled Mushrooms or a batch of cheesey Tortilla Wedges. Or finish with Cherry Cobbler or fresh Apple Pie. Now you can with this good-for-you collection of tantalizing appetizers and desserts. Your mouth will water with every turn of the page, but don't worry: complete nutrition information accompanies every recipe. #CCBGSFF

Nonmember: $8.95; ADA Member: $7.15

Easy & Elegant Entrees

Pull up a chair to Fettucine with Peppers and Broccoli, Pasta with Vegetable Clam Sauce, Steak with Brandied Onions, Baked Chicken with Wine Sauce, and many others. Cooking for a crowd? Try Baked Shrimp Mushroom Casserole. Now you can put all your entrees on the table in minutes, and they're always low in fat and calories. #CCBEEE

Nonmember: $8.95; ADA Member: $7.15

Savory Soups & Salads

Complement those swordfish steaks with the fresh crunch of Zucchini and Carrot Salad. Or savor the exotic tastes of Mediterranean Chicken Salad. Try a bowl of Hot Clam Chowder to warm you up on a cold winter night. Or cool down with the refreshing tang of a bowl of Gazpacho on a scorching summer day. Whether you're in the mood for a little something extra or just a change of pace, you'll find dozens of choices in *Savory Soups & Salads*. #CCBSSS

Nonmember: $8.95; ADA Member: $7.15

Quick & Hearty Main Dishes

Fill up on these delicious main dishes and breakfast foods without blowing your healthy meal plan. Craving pork chops? Choose from Apple Cinnamon Pork Chops, Basil Pork Chops, or Pork Chops Milanese. Denying yourself a hearty breakfast? Try Baked French Toast with Raspberry Sauce, Turkey Sausage, or a Western Omelet. Now you can sit down to delicious, good-for-you main dishes that will satisfy you long after the meal is over. #CCBQHMD

Nonmember: $8.95; ADA Member: $7.15

Simple & Tasty Side Dishes

Turn squash into crunchy morsels of golden goodness with Oven-Fried Yellow Squash. Spice up your eggplant with Tangy Creole Sauce. Taste Rice and Peas Italiano and never be satisfied with plain rice again. Use fresh parsley to create Parsley-Stuffed Potatoes—a truly special side dish. And say goodbye to the ordinary with Tomato and Artichoke Salad, Potato Parmesan Chips, and Golden Vegetable Combo. Now you can learn how to give fresh flavor to all your favorites with the dozens of recipes you'll find in *Simple & Tasty Side Dishes*. #CCBSTSD

Nonmember: $8.95; ADA Member: $7.15

HOW TO ORDER

• • • •

To Order by Phone: just call us at **1-800-ADA-ORDER** and have your credit card ready. VISA, Mastercard, and American Express are accepted. Please mention code CK79602 when ordering.

To Order by Mail: on a separate sheet of paper, write down the books you're ordering and calculate the total using the shipping & handling chart below. (NOTE: Virginia residents add 4.5% sales tax; Georgia residents add 6% sales tax.) Then include your check, written to the American Diabetes Association, with your order and mail to:

American Diabetes Association
Order Fulfillment Department
P.O. BOX 930850
Atlanta, GA 31193-0850

Shipping & Handling Chart

up to $30.00	$30.01–$50.00	over $50.00
add $3.00	add $4.00	add 8%

Allow 2–3 weeks for shipment.
Add $3 to shipping & handling for each extra shipping address.
Add $15 for each overseas shipment.

PRICES SUBJECT TO CHANGE WITHOUT NOTICE.